Mikhail Tomba

Cure the Incurable

First English Edition

Healthy Life Press Inc.

Disclaimer
Any suggestions for techniques, treatments, or lifestyle change described in the book should be used at the reader's discretion under the guidance of a licensed therapist or health-care practitioner. The author, editors, translator and publisher disclaim any and all liability arising directly or indirectly from use of any information contained in this book.

© 2005 by Mikhail Tombak
English version © 2005 by Healthy Life Press Inc.

Translating: Jan Madejski
Cover design: Luke Zukowski

All rights reserved. No part of this book may be reproduced or transmitted in any form or by any means, electronic or mechanical, including photocopying, recording or by any information storage retrieval system, without written permission from the publisher.

Published by:
Healthy Life Press Inc.
1685 H Street PMB 860
Blaine, WA 98230
USA

http://www.starthealthylife.com
info@starthealthylife.com

Tel. (888) 575-3173
Tel. (604) 468-1213

First English Edition

ISBN -10:   0-9727328-3-7
ISBN -13: 978-0-9727328-3-3

LCCN 2005931848

Printed and bound in Poland by
Drukarnia Wydawnictw Naukowych Sp.z o.o., Lodz

Contents

Alcoholism • Anemia • Arrhythmia • Arteriosclerosis • Arthritis • Ascaris (intestinal parasites) • Bloating • Burns • Bone, joint, and muscle pains • Bronchial asthma • Bronchitis • Constipation • Diabetes • Eczema • Eye disorders • Excessive night sweating • Flu • Furuncles (boils) • Fungal infections • Headaches • Heartburn • Hemorrhoids • High blood pressure • Insomnia • Kidney disorders • Lack of appetite (children) • Liver disorders • Low blood pressure • Menopause • Nipple inflammation • Obesity • Swelling • Staphylococcus Aureus infection • Sore throat • Thyroid gland disorders

Spring salads • Summer and fall salads • Winter salads • Sauces and mayonnaises • Cold soups • Desserts

To my readers

Panaceia and Hygieia, daughters of Asklepios, who was the Greek god of medicine and healing (Aesculapius in Roman mythology), varied in their approach to human health. Panaceia (Latin "Panacea") wanted to help people by finding a miraculous potion against all diseases. "Humans don't need to learn about their diseases. It's enough if I am concerned with them," she liked to say. Hygieia (whose name is the source of the word "hygiene") was more interested in the prevention of sickness and the continuation of good health, trying to explain to humans that diseases are a reflection of their unhealthy life style. She advised people to watch and learn from nature, and to live in harmony with her. Both sisters believed they were right, and so they parted, one in search for a miraculous all-curing medication, the other on her quest to educate humans about the principles of healthy life.

When we feel unwell and complain about our heart, stomach, or joints, we tend to look for some external causes. We can usually blame something "out there" and cover up our own neglect and ignorance about basic principles of healthy life style. It's not easy to admit that the real cause is actually "in here."

We are the only ones responsible for our pains, diseases, and premature aging. By leading unhealthy life, we allow our body's vital energy to decrease. Unhealthy diet causes the accumulation of toxins that are difficult to eliminate. They poison us, causing a lot of pain and manifesting themselves as diseases in our organs.

If we were willing to expend some effort, we would be able to live longer and enjoy good health. Unhealthy lifestyle brings premature aging and undue suffering.

I'm strongly convinced that in many health problems, we can be our own doctor and therapist. For that, we need to learn enough about the functioning of our body, in order to identify and eliminate the real causes of our afflictions.

In my practice, I tested many remedies originating from different healing traditions and orientations. The book contains what I selected and believe to be the most valuable from those natural remedies. Please make the best out of it.

Remedies, routines, and recipes presented here don't cause any side effects. If you have any concerns or doubts about using them, please consult a holistically oriented physician, one that sees natural therapies as a valuable addition to conventional medical practice.

Mikhail Tombak

September, 2005

PS   I recommend reading the book three times:

    1. Read the entire text.
    2. Read only the parts that apply to your particular
       situation.
    3. Read only the selected remedies you are going to try.

The doctor of the future will give no medicine, but will interest his patient in the care of the human frame, in diet, and in the cause and prevention of disease.

Thomas Edison

Don't Be Afraid of "Civilization Diseases"

Before we inquire into the causes of "civilization diseases," I would like to present the results of two independent studies, conducted at different locations and time. **They confirm without doubt the wisdom of eastern medicine stating that nobody ever dies of moderation in eating, while overeating is the usual cause of premature death.**

A commission of the World Health Organization did some research in a few Tibetan monasteries. Ninety percent of the monks were examined, some of them very advanced in age. It turned out that the monks, regardless of their age, were physically fit and almost completely healthy. In 60% of the cases there was no tooth decay, circulatory disorders or digestive disorders. Their diet is very modest. They don't have refrigerators or natural gas stoves; they never eat meat, sugar or any refined products. The main items on their menu are barley cakes, herbal tea and clear water. Turnips, carrots, and rice

9

enrich the diet in the summertime.

According to World Health Organization data, in such developed countries as the USA, Germany or France, where the consumption of milk, meat, and refined products is the greatest, the general health level is much worse. In the USA, for example, two families out of three have been touched by cancer, two people out of five suffer and die from heart problems, and many suffer from diabetes. Chronic diseases affect 19% of the population - that's close to one out of every five people.

In Germany, 20% of the population suffers from diabetes, and 20% of the children at the age of eight to sixteen have developmental problems - both physical and intellectual. Rheumatism and joint inflammations affect 15-17% of the people.

In France, allergies affect 15-20% of the population. There are 450 thousand children under 18 with hearing and sight problems, and 1.5 million children aged six and under suffer from asthma. In all highly industrialized countries the number of children born with some kind of health disorder doubled in the last 25 years.

As it turns out, we often use forks and spoons to dig our own graves.

Numerous researches have tried to identify and examine the evasive microbe that is supposed to cause common cold. As recently as in the 1940-ies the scientists explained the ineffectiveness of the research by the fact that the microbe is too small to be seen under the available microscopes. Later spectacular technical advances, including electron microscope, didn't change the situation. Sophisticated optical equipment allowed the discovery of hundreds of new microorganisms, but none of them could be pinned down as the only cause of common cold.

Today, more than 200 different viruses are said to cause the symptoms of the common cold: rhinoviruses, coronaviruses, adenoviruses, coxsackieviruses, echoviruses, orthomyxoviruses (including influenza A and B viruses, which cause flu), paramyxoviruses, enteroviruses, ... the list goes on and on... The causes of 30 to 50 percent of adult colds remain unidentified.

Why can't we identify the microbe that causes the common cold? - Because there is no such thing. Each of the suspected microorganisms is only feeding on the mucus produced in the body suffering from common cold. That mucus, resulting from wrong nutritional habits, is in the body all the time. In the spring and fall seasons, the body starts cleaning itself of the excess amounts of mucus. That's when germs show up and start dissolving and then destroying or removing the mucus, in effect helping us to clean up our body. What do we do then? We take medications to get rid of the microbes. This way, we end up killing what is helping us and allowing the mucus to stay in our body. After some time, we get sick again either with common cold or influenza. The root of the problem remains the same, only this time a different kind of microorganism is feeding on the mucus.

Year after year in spring and fall seasons, epidemic numbers of people suffer from runny noses, bone aches, and other common cold symptoms. We have more and more medications intended to kill the microbes. The germs, tiny as they are, are not stupid. They want to live, and they find ways to become immune to our drugs. It doesn't take a prophet to predict the result of such "wars". The stronger and more effective drugs we invent the more vicious microbes we have to deal with. Who is the loser in this war? Our health is. All drugs, even those considered very safe, cause side effects.

What then is the cause of common cold? It is waste accumulated in our body. If our ability to discard that waste is deficient, the large intestine becomes a warehouse for all this filth. From there, it's distributed to the whole body and forms unhealthy mucus. When the amount of toxic mucus becomes

11

dangerous, our body tries to clean itself through the nose, and this becomes what we call common cold. As viruses and bacteria invade the mucus, they bring about inflammations and fever. These are facts that deserve some thought.

To convince you that many of our diseases are caused by improper diet, I'd like to reflect on the longevity record of Hunza Valley inhabitants in India. The average longevity among 32,000 inhabitants is 120 years. What is their secret?

Sir Robert McCarrison - a Scottish physician who lived in Hunza Valley area for 15 years - concluded that the main factor in the inhabitants' longevity is their diet. They are vegetarians and their usual diet consists of raw fruits and vegetables in the summer; in the winter it consists mainly of grain sprouts, dried apricots, and sheep cheese.

On his return home McCarrison conducted a series of experiments with animals, in order to be finally convinced about the connection between diet and longevity. One group of animals was fed the diet of a typical London family (white bread, herrings, refined sugar, canned and cooked vegetables, etc. It resulted in various "human" disorders among the animals. The other group of animals, fed a "Hunza Valley diet," remained healthy throughout the experiments.

It is believed that climate influences longevity. It is an interesting fact that other groups of people living in similar climates to that of Hunza Valley suffer from many health disorders and their longevity is two times shorter. The mountain climate does not prevent them from diseases because their diet is unhealthy.

In contrast to neighboring ethnic groups, Hunza Valley inhabitants look very much like Caucasians. Historians propose a theory that merchants and soldiers who settled in Hunza Valley during the expedition of Alexander the Great along the Indus River started the tribal communities there. That means even Caucasians can live long if they eat properly.

"All diseases enter our body through the mouth," said Hippocrates. This brilliant observation is a few thousand years old, but we haven't been willing to use it yet. I often wonder why. Did he not say it loud enough for people to take notice? In any case, generation after generation passes down to their children poor nutritional habits, and along with those habits they pass down many health problems. As an excuse, we say that times are hard and the progress of civilization puts a heavy burden on us. However, we are rather burdened by our excess weight, laziness, and complete disregard for the physiological rules by which our body functions. **We know how to deal with complicated economic issues, how to use computers, or how to repair an electronic instrument with thousands of connections, but we cannot answer the simple question about the number of times we urinate in a day or about the color of our urine.** In order to understand what is good and what is harmful for us we need to watch the way our body functions. That is the basic rule in good health maintenance.

*Human body is designed in accordance
with the laws of physics and chemistry.
These laws never change. They are
recorded in every nerve and every muscle.
They organize cells, tissues and organs by
assigning to them specific functions.*

Your Fighting Chance Against Osteoporosis

As winter begins many elderly people get anxious. They worry about cold, snow, and slippery sidewalks. The risk of falling and breaking a bone is very real. Persons suffering from osteoporosis are particularly prone to bone fractures.

Based on statistics, the most dangerous are fractures in the area of the hip joint. This brings permanent disability in about half of all cases. In developed countries, osteoporosis starts placing itself near the top of all "civilization diseases". It used to be the common opinion that this disease attacks mostly women. Present research shows that it affects men and women to the same degree. Moreover, children as young as 8-11 are now diagnosed more frequently. For most inhabitants of big cities, the first symptoms of osteoporosis can be usually noticed at the age of 30.

What is osteoporosis? Why do strong and healthy bones become weak and prone to fractures or shattering?

Osteoporosis means calcium deficiency in the bones. As we

know, the main ingredient of the bone tissue is calcium. If for some reason our body is deficient in calcium, our bones become porous and start resembling Swiss cheese.

According to conventional medicine, osteoporosis is an incurable disease with a genetic component. Medicine doesn't really know how to treat genetic diseases. This means such diagnosis leaves only slim chances of being cured. The best we can do is to stop the disease's progression. To achieve that, specialists recommend drinking more milk and eating more cheese. The usual advice for men is to reduce the consumption of alcohol and tobacco and to take formulas containing synthetic calcium and vitamin D3. Women get the same advice plus estrogen therapy.

Medical practice proves that formulas containing calcium and hormones can delay the development of the disease. However, most specialists I know agree, that complete cure is impossible. It's not up to me to evaluate the effectiveness of existing therapies. Dozens of research institutes, all over the world, inquire into the causes of osteoporosis and its treatment. One thing is certain - presently available therapies focus on delivering more calcium to the body and forcing the body to assimilate that extra calcium.

At a seminar dealing with healthy lifestyle, a woman told me a very sad story. Her bones are weak even though she drinks 1-1.5qt (1-1.5L) of milk a day throughout all her life, milk-based soups and grains are part of her diet every other day, and she takes large amounts of calcium and vitamin C whenever she catches a cold. In other words, her body is supplied more calcium than it needs. Despite all that, when she broke her arm, the bone wouldn't heal. That's when she was diagnosed with osteoporosis.

Some readers who eat plenty of dairy products and regularly take calcium pills are probably surprised to be diagnosed with osteoporosis, or calcium deficiency. Why does this happen?

The form of calcium we get from pasteurized and skimmed milk, synthetic formulas, pills, and other such sources, goes through our body without being assimilated. The bones get practically nothing from that kind of calcium. Every time when increased amounts of calcium are needed for life processes (e.g. when the weather changes), our blood takes the extra amount from the bones. This is why people often complain about bone aches when the weather is about to change. Supplying our body with hard-to-assimilate form of calcium is like spinning wheels when our car is stuck in snow - the faster we spin the wheels the deeper they dig in. The engine works at full power and wastes lots of fuel, but we don't get anywhere.

Two forms of calcium

There are two forms of calcium in our food products. Organic calcium - easily assimilated into our bones - is found in vegetables, fruits (especially in the peel), freshly squeezed juices, eggs, bran, wheat and oat sprouts, nuts, honey, and fresh cow or goat milk. Non-organic and hard-to-assimilate form of calcium is contained in all refined products, bread, pasteurized or cooked milk and their products, boiled water; all products processed in temperatures over 212F(100C) (cooked, fried, etc.), and synthetically produced calcium formulas. If our diet consists mainly of refined food products, pasteurized or boiled milk, crunchy bread, cooked or fried products, and if the water we use is usually boiled (this is true for many people), it is obvious why our bones are so often affected by osteoporosis.

Organic calcium forms in our body easily-dissolvable salts that are essential for circulatory processes. These salts protect our blood from bacteria getting in through blood vessels, play a part in the healthy growth of bones and teeth, enhance the functioning of our nervous system, increase immunity, and have many other useful functions.

Non-organic form of calcium is only used to a small degree in the bone growth. It mainly serves as the material to form hard-to-dissolve calcium salts that become the core of kidney, liver, and gallbladder stones. People who like fresh white bread and rolls (these products are the main source of non-organic calcium) put themselves at risk of calcium stones, especially in the gallbladder. In order to assimilate non-organic calcium, the body has to draw on its reserves of micro- and macro-elements, which has a negative effect on other physiological processes.

Some impatient readers may wonder why I provide so much detail. It would seem to be enough to simply give some advice on what to eat and what to avoid. Simple doesn't necessarily mean effective. Each of us is a unique individuality and there is no universal remedy against osteoporosis. This and all other diseases can only be defeated if we have enough understanding to find the weaknesses of our "opponent". A detailed description of all processes linked with calcium assimilation, and of all our common nutritional mistakes, helps develop such understanding.

We need to understand that our body is a complex system in which all cells are connected by countless interactions. This is why only a complex approach affecting all vital organs and systems is able to cure every health problem regardless of its specific location - in our bones, heart, liver, or in the big toe of our right foot.

What causes calcium deficiency

Among the different elements in our body, the amount of calcium is the fifth after the four basic elements: carbon, oxygen, hydrogen, and nitrogen. On the average, there is about 2.6lb (1.2kg) of calcium in a human body and 99% of this amount is contained in the bones.

There are two processes taking place in our bone tissue:

1. Breakdown, accompanied by the release of calcium and phosphorus to the blood
2. Rebuilding by fresh deposits of calcium salts

In one day, up to 700mg of calcium is released from the bone tissue of an adult, and the same amount of fresh calcium should be deposited again. The whole skeletal system of growing children is completely rebuilt in 1-2 years, in adults the same process takes 10-12 years.

Besides supporting our body (keeping in the vertical position), the bone tissue has the function of storing calcium and phosphorus, so that the body can have an emergency supply of these elements when it does not get an adequate amount from the food we eat. The calcium level in our blood is consistent. Even in the last stages of osteoporosis, the blood can maintain 99.9% of the required level by taking calcium from the bones. If our blood has to take calcium from the bones day after day, the bone mass starts diminishing.

It's known that products such as meat, cheese, sugar, and animal fats produce large amounts of harmful acids (lactic, oxalic, uric, and other) when they are digested. Calcium salts are used to neutralize these acids and protect our body from poisoning. The more of such products we eat the less calcium is left in our bones.

Sugar - the worst enemy of calcium

One of the main causes of calcium deficiency is high consumption of sugar and products containing sugar. It is a synthetic substance and its digestion results in many poisonous acids in our body. Huge amounts of mineral salts, containing mostly calcium, are needed to neutralize these acids. Where are they taken from? They are taken from our bones and teeth, where they are found in the highest concentration. We develop a taste for sweets from early childhood and even adults consume hundreds of times more sugar than the safe amount every day. It's obvious why children suffer from tooth decay, adults from gum disease, and the bones of the elderly are as porous as Swiss cheese (osteoporosis). Is osteoporosis a genetic disease? I would say no. Our bad habits are rather the thing passed down from generation to generation to cause diseases.

In conclusion, one of the main causes of osteoporosis is our excessive liking for sweets. I often hear parents say: "How can I refuse my child a candy. Childhood should be sweet". I would advise parents to think more about providing a healthy and happy childhood for their offspring. When the children grow old, little pleasures of their sweet childhood may cost them years of suffering from bone and spine pains.

Recent research discovered three main principles of calcium assimilation:

1. Calcium is flushed out of the body when there is excess or deficiency of fats.
2. Excess or deficiency in phosphorus or magnesium has negative effect on calcium assimilation.
3. The content of Vitamin D in food products is important for calcium assimilation.

These discoveries explain why people who drink pasteurized or cooked milk don't get as much calcium in their body as they imagine.

I'd like to say a little bit more about milk because typical a large part of our diet consists of milk products. Those readers who've read the chapter "Addiction to milk" in my first book ("Can We Live 150 Years?" page 20) know my opinion about this issue. If you wish to continue drinking milk anyway, drink it as fresh as possible and only from cows that graze on ecologically clean pastures. This would have some health benefits, but most people don't have access to such milk. Our body assimilates calcium fully when the proportion of calcium to phosphorus in the product is 1 to 1.3, and the proportion of calcium to magnesium is 1 to 0.5. In pasteurized or cooked milk these proportions are 1 to 0.7 and 1 to 0.1. On top of that, 40-60% of Vitamin D is destroyed in the process of pasteurization. This way 80-90% of calcium contained in pasteurized milk isn't assimilated. What does our body get from drinking pasteurized milk? It gets casein (hard to digest protein, used in industry as raw material for glue manufacturing), animal fat that causes high cholesterol levels, and radioactive isotope Strontium 90 that participates in the formation of cancer cells. Milk is recently often described as "silent killer". I fully support this point of view.

Doctors participating in an international congress on the impact of living and work environment on health were surprised to find out that Europeans were deficient in 900mg of calcium a day. Ninety percent of their calcium intake comes from milk and its products. The inhabitants of India, Chile, South Africa, and Turkey need only 300mg of calcium intake a day. Dairy products are only 10% of their diet while the rest is grains, vegetables, fruits, nuts, and sprouts. These findings don't surprise me. All substances needed for calcium assimilation are found in natural food products in ideal proportions. Those proportions are disturbed in processed foods, especially in pasteurized milk.

Based on these facts, we can conclude that the habit of drinking cow milk - formed from early childhood and passed down from generation to generation - results in serious calcium deficiency. The damage done by milk consumption is hundreds of times greater than any benefits derived from it.

Vitamin D - an ally of calcium

The main function of Vitamin D is regulating calcium exchange in our body. Our kidneys turn Vitamin D into a compound that supports the assimilation of calcium. Vitamin C also plays an important part in that reaction. Both Vitamin D and Vitamin C are therefore essential for calcium assimilation by our skeletal system.

Food products alone cannot provide adequate amounts of Vitamin D. Eggs are one of the main food products containing Vitamin D. They are not usually recommended due to high fat content and resulting high cholesterol levels - an opinion I definitely disagree with. Butter is another good source, but it's often replaced by synthetic margarine, which releases Vitamin D with great difficulty. Liver and fish are also rich in Vitamin D. However, we don't usually eat them raw. Thermal processing lives only tiny amounts of Vitamin D in these products.

Vitamin D is sometimes called "sun vitamin" because it is created in the body under the influence of ultraviolet rays. We have been told for some time to avoid sunlight because it increases the possibility of getting cancers. Sunlight is blamed as the biggest culprit in many health problems. Many experts re-

peat the warning: "Avoid sunlight - it damages your health."
We are forgetting that sun energy is essential for everything
that's alive on this planet.

Let's talk about sunlight, focusing not on its potential hazards but on health benefits we can receive from it. Our body
produces Vitamin D under the influence of sunrays. The main
function of this vitamin is facilitating calcium assimilation. It's
also essential for blood coagulation, normal growth of bones
and other tissue, and the functioning of our heart and nervous
system.

Deficiency in Vitamin D (due to inadequate exposure to sunlight) strongly impairs metabolic processes and causes poor
functioning of blood vessels. They are not able to prevent bacteria from getting into our blood, which weakens our body's
defense mechanisms. We become more sensible to weather
changes and more prone to infections. This way, our general
health level is in danger due to inadequate amounts of Vitamin
D and resulting deficiency in calcium and its salts.

Both Vitamin D and calcium are always available in pharmacies in the form of pills, but it's very difficult to establish
proper doses because demand can be very different for different individuals. We have to realize that either excess of or
deficiency in Vitamin D impairs calcium assimilation. This is
why pills can cause more damage than good.

We cannot rely on food we eat or formulas we take in assu-
ring adequate supply of Vitamin D. It has to be produced by our
own body in a natural way - under the influence of sunlight.

Our primal ancestors who spent most of their lives under the
open sky didn't suffer from Vitamin D deficiency. Some primi-
tive tribes existing today aren't affected by it, either. It mostly
affects people living in cities where the amount of sunlight getting into their dwellings through windows is very low.

We should remember that sunlight exposure should happen in small doses, 20-30 minutes a day. Use it for its health benefits not for an attractive suntan.

Research proves that the best time for sunbathing is in the morning - between sunrise and 10 a.m. Between 10 a.m. and 5 p.m. the sunrays are too intensive and burn our skin, leading to its premature aging. Japanese professor Nishi found out that certain water and aerobic exercises can stimulate the production of Vitamin D in our body. This is why it would be beneficial to acquire the habit of daily alternate hot-and-cold showers in the morning and the evening. Regular use of sauna also helps in the synthesis of Vitamin D.

When we get a dark suntan, the production of Vitamin D becomes slower. This is why, as our skin darkens, it's better to spend more time in the shade.

When you are on holidays and get a dark suntan, eat more eggs, butter, liver, fish, fruits and vegetables. They are all good sources of Vitamin D.

Sunshine is a priceless gift from nature. When used wisely, its energy is beneficial for our health.

There is another important fact about Vitamin D. It is found in our skin glands. The more we wash our skin with the use of artificial cosmetic products the more of the vitamin we wash out of our body. This doesn't mean we have to give up hygiene. After we use synthetic products to wash our skin, it's a good idea to rub some natural vegetable oil in it - if not on the entire body, at least on our hands and feet because that's where the synthesis of Vitamin D mainly happens. It's even better to prepare the oil by adding two handfuls of rose flakes to a bottle containing 7 oz (200g) of vegetable oil and leaving it in a dark place for seven days. The bottle can be kept handy and used after washing dishes, doing laundry, etc. Our skin acts as a double filter - it discards toxins from our body and absorbs useful substances from the environment.

I hope that this discussion helps the reader understand the qualities of Vitamin D and the fact that our modern lifestyle causes its deficiency, resulting in incomplete assimilation of calcium.

Now I'd like to present some important facts about **Vitamin C.** It is also essential for maintaining good health. No oxidation reaction can happen without Vitamin C and we would die, defenseless against viruses that constantly attack our body. Our blood vessels would be unable to circulate blood - they would turn into a system of empty tubes.

You will find more information about the qualities of Vitamin C later in this book. At this time, I would like to focus not on its role in the functioning of our body, but on its physical and chemical properties.

Unfortunately Vitamin C is a very volatile substance. It disintegrates under the influence of direct sunlight or even regular daylight; cooking in temperatures over 212F(100C) also destroys it. For example, cooking vegetable soup destroys 50% of Vitamin C, and leaving the soup on the stove for another three hours causes it to lose another 20%. If we let it stand for another six hours or warm it up again, it practically loses all its Vitamin C content. By peeling potatoes, we get rid of 30% of their Vitamin C content, by cooking them - another 30-40%. This way, if we mainly eat cooked food and on top of that warm it up a few times, we get only minimal amounts of Vitamin C from it.

Luckily, we can fill this gap by eating fruits and vegetables, which contain a lot of Vitamin C. The benefits of eating raw fruits and vegetables have been discovered rather late. Earlier (starting from 1960-ies) such diet wasn't recommended - especially for the elderly - because a lot of people experienced some form of digestive system disorders. The elderly had difficulty eating raw fruits and vegetables anyway because of poor condition of their teeth. To prevent stomach disorders, people avoided raw fruits and vegetables or at least peeled them to get rid of stomach-damaging nitrates. However, the peel also contains most calcium. Higher consumption of milk and meat was recommended. Ironically, the more animal protein is consumed the more Vitamin C is necessary for our body...

I'd like to mention another shocking fact about Vitamin C. Research proved that one cigarette destroys 25mg of Vitamin C in our body - a quarter of normal daily demand. This way, smoking totally wipes out Vitamin C content in our body. It's enough to have one smoker in the family - the rest will suffer these consequences through passive smoking, especially those who passively inhale from early childhood. Vitamin C makes us immune against colds. There are epidemic numbers of flu and common cold cases every spring and fall. It suggests that we are highly deficient in this vitamin.

What about vitamin pills? Not only vitamin C - all synthetic vitamins in the form of pills are harmful. First, most vitamins are compounds formed by plants in the process of biosynthesis under the influence of sunlight. Vitamins in plants are in forms (pro-vitamins) that are easily assimilated by the human body. Plants also contain all mineral salts and other compounds (some still unknown) that help in full assimilation of vitamins.

Second, artificial vitamins are non-organic crystalloid substances treated as foreign by our body. They are assimilated with difficulty or not assimilated at all (especially in the case of metabolic disorders). This is why many people notice that their urine has the same color and smell as the vitamins. There are frequent cases of rejection in the form of nausea, weakness, or itching.

Third, one of the side effects of taking synthetic vitamins is increased appetite. This happens because the body, in order to assimilate the vitamins, needs additional amounts of mineral salts, carbohydrates, and proteins. Unlike plant-based foods, synthetic vitamins do not have these ingredients, and the body instinctively looks for more food, which leads to obesity.

In most people's mind, vitamin C has the opinion of a harmless supplement. However, in recent years physicians started noticing more side effects that are caused by vitamin C overdosing. It is common that people take vitamin C in liberal amounts, sometimes 0.14-0.21oz (4-6g) a day, as a remedy against flu and some viral infections, while the recommended amount is about 100mg a day.

Scientists in many countries agree with the opinion that taking synthetic vitamin C does not increase immunity against colds, and its large doses make the symptoms of some infectious-allergic diseases (especially rheumatism) more severe.

The most dangerous effect of high doses of vitamin C is increased coagulability of blood, leading to blood clots. Another side effect can be formation of stones from oxalic acid and uric acid in our kidneys and bladder.

Synthetic vitamin C destroys other vitamins. This is why patients who get shots of vitamin B2 are advised by physicians to stop taking vitamin C during that time.

Large doses of vitamin C interfere with the production of insulin by the pancreas in diabetics and cause an increase of sugar level in their urine and blood. Recent research shows that vitamin C overdosing slows the transmission of nerve-muscle impulses, causing increased muscle fatigue and lowering the coordination between eyes and muscles.

It is a good idea to consult your physician about the effects of synthetic vitamin C. Natural vitamins found in large amounts in fruits and vegetables are most beneficial - it's not possible to overdose them.

The biggest factor interfering with proper calcium exchange in our body might be our liking for white flour products. They contain large amounts of calcium in hard-to-assimilate form. This kind of calcium forms durable and insoluble compounds with some acids (oxalic and uric acid). Frequent pains in our spine, joints and muscles are no surprise if we consider that bread and other white-flour products are the basis of our diet.

How are insoluble calcium salts formed in our body

Most of us eat too much. That results from eating more out of habit than hunger. We were convinced in our childhood that we have to eat a few meals a day regardless of how we feel. Our body is overwhelmed by the necessity to digest, process, and assimilate excessive amounts of food. Large amounts of acids are produced as a result of eating animal proteins. These acids together with calcium form insoluble crystalloid toxic compounds. Our body is unable to remove them and they start forming deposits in our joints. It's a slow process, taking many years. Most people don't notice anything until their joints start giving trouble. Nature provided our joints with the means to be flexible in the form of a special substance, a kind of lubricant. The amount of that lubricant does not decrease by itself, no matter the age. When insoluble calcium compounds start pushing the lubricant out and "cementing" our joints, we experience pain, decreased range of motion, and lack of flexibility.

Our legs are the first targets of the "attack". They have the highest number of bones, compared to other parts of our body (there are 26 bones in our foot). Toxic crystals move up from our feet, causing pain in the knees. Then they move up to lumbar joints. As years go by, salt crystals move even higher along the spine - to our neck, shoulders, elbows, even fingers. Getting up in the morning, we complain about all kinds of joint pains. We can hear grinding sounds when turning our head. Some people have trouble closing their fists.

We tend to blame it all on aging but when we watch younger people, we often find that they too have problems with joint flexibility. Children don't spend enough time actively playing outdoors. They spend too much time sitting in front of computers and don't get enough physical exercise to keep their bones and joints healthy. The less time we spend being physically active the higher our risk of becoming ill with osteoporosis.

The most likely factors contributing to the risk of osteoporosis, based on the observation of patients, (including those who were cured) are the following:

1. Deficiency in vitamins D and C
2. Diet rich in thermally processed products
3. Using mainly boiled water
4. Not enough fruits, vegetables, and their freshly squeezed juices in the diet
5. Eating fruits and vegetables without peel
6. Improperly prepared meals (long cooking and frying)
7. Overeating
8. Smoking
9. Lack of exercise
10. High consumption of milk
11. High consumption of bread and other flour-based products
12. High consumption of sugar and sweets
13. High consumption of animal fats
14. Taking large amounts of synthetic vitamins
15. Eating refined products containing insoluble (non-organic) calcium: pre-cooked grains, pasta, ready-made soups and other

After honestly considering all of the above points, many would probably have to put a checkmark next to each of them. This would mean for them a high probability of becoming ill with osteoporosis.

To summarize, we bring osteoporosis on ourselves by our unhealthy lifestyle. We also pass it down to our children. The problem is not in our genes but our bad habits that result in osteoporosis and other "civilization diseases".

To effectively fight osteoporosis, we have to eat a lot of fruits and vegetables and to drink their juices. The most beneficial are the ones with high content of calcium, Vitamins C and D, phosphorus, potassium, and magnesium (see table below and salad recipes pages 215-220).

Table 1.

Food products rich in microelements and vitamins

Calcium	Phosphorus	Potassium	Magnesium	Vitamin C	Vitamin D
Fruit and vegetable peel	Green peas	Spinach	Cabbage	Tomatoes	Tomatoes
	Spinach	Cucumbers	Carrot	Carrot	Carrot
Bran	Nuts	Potatoes	Beets	Lettuce	Cabbage
Horse bean	Oats	Carrot	Lettuce	Spinach	Potatoes
Spinach	Horse bean	Onion	Oats	Cabbage	Turnip
Carrot	Rye	Parsley	Barley	Potatoes	Beets
Turnip	Barley	Asparagus	Wheat	Beets	Spinach
Lettuce	Wheat		Spinach	Apples	Horse bean
Green pees	Cucumbers		Parsley	Cranberries	Green pees
Dandelion	Cabbage		Dandelion	Green peas	Dandelion
Celery	Cauliflower		Nettle	Currants	
Apples	Apples			Gooseberry	
Cherries	Pears			Raspberry	
Gooseberry				Parsley	
Wild strawberries				Nettle	

Remedies against osteoporosis

Eggshells are not trash. They are helpful in the treatment of osteoporosis. They are an ideal source of calcium that is in 90% assimilated by our bones. Besides calcium carbonate, eggshells contain all the microelements essential for our body: copper, fluorine, iron, manganese, molybdenum, sulfur, silicon, zinc, and other - 27 elements in total. The composition of an eggshell is very similar to that of our bones and teeth. German and Hungarian scientists who researched the influence of eggshell therapy on the human body concluded that for both children and adults it had positive results against breaking nails and hair, bleeding gums, constipation, hypersensitivity, insomnia, chronic colds, and asthma. The therapy strengthens the bone tissue and removes radioactive elements from the body.

Eggshell therapy offers invaluable benefits in the treatment and prevention of osteoporosis, without causing any side effects. The therapy is simple and doesn't require any expenses.

Remedy #1
Immerse an eggshell in boiling water for 5 minutes, let it dry, and grind it in a coffee grinder. Take 0.009-0.018oz (0.5-1g) a day. You can mix it with juice squeezed from one half of a lemon or add it to your grains and cottage cheese for osteoporosis prevention. Use this therapy for 30 days twice a year (January and November).

Remedy #2
Juice from black radish leaves is a very effective remedy for children and adults against the abnormal softening of tooth and bone tissue (osteomalacia). For best effects, use a blend of juices squeezed from turnip leaves (3.2oz/90g), dandelions (3.2oz/90g), and carrots (9.9oz/280g) for two servings

31

- in the morning and the evening.

Remedy #3 (Using black radish for body cleansing)

This remedy helps not only in slowing osteoporosis but also in removing excessive amounts of salts from the entire skeletal system. Take 22lb (10kg) of black radish, wash them well (for the purpose of disinfection, you can soak it in a potassium manganiane solution for 15-30 minutes and then rinse well), cut out all fibers and unhealthy spots without peeling. Put the black radish through a juicer - you will get about 3 quarts (3L) of juice. Filter the juice a few times and pour into glass bottles, close the bottles, wrap into dark cloth and store refrigerated (Note: This is important - do not store any other way!). Take 1.05oz (30g) three times a day, independently of your meal times. Do not overdose - this may have dangerous consequences. To achieve expected results, continue the therapy until the entire amount of juice from 22lb (10kg) is finished.

Avoid entirely buns, fatty products, meat, and eggs during the therapy. Stick to plant-based foods.

I would like to warn that people with lots of unhealthy deposits in the skeletal system might experience bone pain, sometimes quite intensive. Don't be afraid and don't take painkillers. Simply continue the therapy. This phenomenon is normal during the cleansing process. A successful therapy can free you from much pain in the future.

Taking baths with added hay extract is very beneficial during black radish juice therapy. Such baths are also recommended at any other time because they rejuvenate the body, calm the nervous system, cleanse the lymphatic system, stop bone and muscle pains, clear skin pores, and improve blood circulation.

Remedy #4

Put a pack of hay (available in pet stores) in a 5qt (5L) pot, pour 3qt (3L) of boiling water on it, cover with a lid, and boil on low heat for 1,5-2 hours. Prepare a bath 113-122 F (45-50C) hot and pour the hay extract in it. Prepare a sheet of plastic foil, large enough to cover your bathtub, and cut in it an opening for your head. Get in the bath and put the cover on tightly to allow as little air exchange as possible (The cover is there to keep ethereal oils from evaporating and allow them to be absorbed by the pores in your skin.) Take a 15-20 minute bath every day or every other day (10-12 baths in total).

Let us sum up all steps you should undertake if you are ill with osteoporosis:

1. Change your diet - avoid products that flush calcium out of your bones (coffee, animal fats, etc.)
2. Drink freshly squeezed fruit juices (at least two glasses a day).
3. Make sure your diet contains an adequate amount of natural vitamins (particularly vitamins C and D).
4. Eat one ground eggshell, one soft-boiled egg, and one apple every day.
5. Regularly eat beans, peas, broccoli, and oats - they all are rich in estrogens.
6. Take alternate hot and cold showers in the morning and the evening.
7. Strengthen your bones by daily exercise (for example, dance and jump to the sounds of your favorite music for 10-15 minutes).
8. Cleanse your body periodically, using cleansing routines presented in this book and in my other book, "Can We Live 150 Years?" (p. 182-210)

Uric Acid - Silent Killer

God created food and the devil created a chef. We seem to forget this old saying. We like eating so much that indulgence became a habit if not an addiction, taking away our ability for rational thinking. Our body can't keep up with the necessity to process excessive amounts of food. We force it to store undigested food remains in various corners of our body. Over the years they decompose and poison us from within, causing diseases and premature aging.

Stomach capacity is different for different individuals. We can roughly determine our proper physiological stomach capacity by joining our palms to form a ball. A meal should not be bigger than half the volume of that ball, and the amount of fluids we drink at a time shouldn't amount to more than a quarter of the ball. Whatever goes over these volumes is excessive and has to be stored. Even if daily amounts of excess food are not large, they accumulate as time goes by.

Almost all our chronic diseases originate from the accumulation of uric acid, which gradually, like rust, eats up our health. Where does it come from? First, it's the result of excessive eating in general; second, from eating too much protein foods (meat, milk, deli, etc.)

Normal blood content of uric acid is very low. When its content increases above normal, uric acid binds with certain blood components and forms gels that clog blood vessels. Blood circulation in those places slows or stops completely. Usually vessels that are the tiniest and most remote from the heart are affected (in hands and legs). Those places (hands and legs) feel unusually cold due to decreased blood circulation. This may result in extreme impairment of blood circulation.

Disorders of our joints and bones, back pains, chronic rheumatism, arthritis, podagra, etc., are caused by excess of uric acid in our body. We are going to suffer in pain as long as its hard crystals are stuck in our bones and muscles. Those suffering from rheumatism or podagra have to understand: to get rid of pain they've been suffering from for years, they need to interrupt the process of uric acid formation and dissolve its deposits accumulated in joints and muscles.

Remedies suggested below helped many people cure conditions that were immobilizing them. One of those people was my mother, a physician with 45 years of experience. She had suffered badly from rheumatism for 30 years until she was willing to try good advice of alternative medicine. The presence of uric acid causes different sets of symptoms, identified as some common health conditions.

Podagra (Gout)

It usually attacks joints in our great toes, less often in the thumbs. Excruciating gouty pains are the usual symptoms. Deposits of crystals cause pain, swelling, and redness in the joint area. Salts deposited by blood form growths that deform our joints and interfere with their mobility. If the deposits of acid keep growing, thick cement-like layers of salt cover the entire joints and prevent them from almost any movement. The illness usually first demonstrates itself with slight pain and decreased mobility in the attacked joints, especially after a longer period of inactivity (e.g. sleep or sitting).

Chronic rheumatism

Chronic rheumatism should be distinguished from acute rheumatism, which is a complication from cold or flu. Chronic rheumatism is related to podagra because both are the result of accumulated uric acid deposits. It seldom affects young people. Older people pay that price for all generous meals in their lifetime.

We can say that rheumatism is a mirror where our bad nutritional habits are reflected. Chronic rheumatism causes swellings and growths that look very much like those in podagra cases, but it isn't as painful as podagra. Its cause is slow metabolism originating from excess of uric acid due to consuming products containing it, or consuming a lot of alcohol, coffee, tea, sweets, and cigarettes.

Anemia

Low count of red blood cells is probably related to high consumption of cooked and refined foods, sugar, animal proteins, and pasteurized milk. Hard-to-assimilate form of calcium forms insoluble salts with uric acid, which results in changing blood composition.

Liver and kidney stones

Uric acid is deposited not only in our joints and muscles but also in kidneys and bile. Salts formed from uric acid and non-organic calcium crystallize in our liver and kidneys. Those crystals are first found in the form of sand, which can squeeze through ducts. Given enough time, stones are formed and result in acute pain (colic) in the liver or kidneys. Sensation of pain while urinating is the first signal of sand formation. However, we usually ignore such signals and don't pay attention until stones are formed and we suffer from severe pain attacks.

Skin conditions

Deposits of uric acid and its salts in our tissues are also the cause of many skin conditions, especially the ones localized in a limited area (e.g. eczema).

Diabetes and obesity

Uric acid is a toxin and our body has to deplete its own resources in order to neutralize it. Normal metabolism is slowed down because minerals, vitamins, macro- and microelements are involved in the process. This leads to disturbing our body's sugar economy (diabetes). As a rule, the next consequence is disturbed fat exchange and abnormal accumulation of fat. This is why many diabetics suffer from obesity.

Neurological diseases

Since uric acid is in direct contact with our blood, its effects aren't limited to our joints, tissues, and muscles. Our brain and nerve centers are also negatively affected by its toxicity. High blood pressure, headaches, migraines, neurasthenia, insomnia, even epilepsy may originate from a common cause - toxic properties of uric acid salts.

I once had a female patient suffering from headaches so terrible that the strongest painkillers couldn't give her any relief. I recommended two things: giving up meat and using a cleansing routine to eliminate uric acid from her body. A month later she didn't have to worry about headaches anymore. Her daughter and friends also started using the same remedy. I've recommended it to many people over the years and they report not only relief from headaches but also from other discomforts such as aches in their joints, bones, and muscles.

Cleansing routine eliminating uric acid from our body

The routine can be used in cases of osteoporosis, podagra (gout), chronic rheumatism, gallbladder and kidney stones, anemia, some neurological disorders, diabetes, obesity, high blood pressure, gastritis, and liver disorders. The best method to get rid of toxic uric acid poisoning our body is to use regular lemon juice. The therapy doesn't require change of climate (often recommended in cases of chronic rheumatism), is relatively inexpensive, and brings fantastic results.

All you need is regular lemons, preferably with thin peel

39

because they contain more juice. Fresh lemon juice quickly changes its composition under the influence of air and sunlight. That's why you need to prepare a new portion every time.

There is a common opinion, especially among people who don't tolerate sour taste very well, that a large amount of lemon juice can cause stomach irritation. There is no basis for such concerns if we understand physiological processes happening in the digestive tract. The taste itself changes in our mouth from sour to sweet under the influence of enzymes. Citric and ascorbic acids that get to the stomach are much weaker than hydrochloric acid contained in gastric juices - they cannot cause any damage to the mucous membrane lining our stomach. Quite the opposite - people suffering from gastritis or ulceration often benefit from lemon juice therapy. Lemon juice is rich in vitamin C, microelements and hormones. It wonderfully cleans insoluble salts and slime out of our body. **Drinking juice squeezed from one lemon every day helps us stay young.** It also contains estrogen-like phytochemical substances and therefore is very beneficial for older females. Some chemical compounds found in lemon juice are very effective in the prevention of infectious diseases. We should drink lemon juice as a preventative measure against the flu epidemic and colds in late fall and early spring.

Lemon juice can be used in a preventative or a healing therapy.

Remedy #5
Preventative lemon therapy

Use the following amounts of lemon juice:

Day 1 - 1 lemon - Day 10
Day 2 - 2 lemons - Day 9

Day 3 - 3 lemons - Day 8
Day 4 - 4 lemons - Day 7
Day 5 - 5 lemons - Day 6

From the first to the fifth day, we add one lemon every day and from the sixth to the tenth day, we subtract one lemon a day. In total, we drink juice squeezed from 30 lemons during ten days.

Lemon juice can be prepared in the following way:

Cut a lemon horizontally in half, squeeze both halves and drink the juice without adding any sugar. If you are not able to drink pure lemon juice, dilute it with water and add one teaspoon of honey. You should not discard the squeezed lemon - it contains valuable phytochemical ingredients and essential oils that are beneficial for the heart, blood vessels, and brain. Cut the squeezed lemon into small pieces, put them in a jar, add honey or sugar, and put in the refrigerator. In ten hours, you will have an excellent lemon extract that can be mixed with boiled or mineral water and used instead of tea or coffee.

Healing lemon therapy

Use only pure lemon juice for the purpose of this therapy - do not dilute it with water; do not add any honey or sugar. It should be prepared the same way as for preventative lemon therapy. You can drink it half an hour before or one hour after your meals, whichever is more convenient. To treat serious, chronic diseases, we have to drink in total juice squeezed from 200 lemons during the therapy. This number might surprise you. Some people get a sensation of sour taste in their mouth just by thinking about such amount of citric acid. This is not an error - it has to be at least 200 lemons (more is allowed).

In the course of my practice, I have seen hundreds of people who enjoyed good health thanks to drinking large amounts of lemon juice. I drank up to ten cups of lemon juice (squeezed from about forty lemons) daily. When you try, you will find out that there is nothing to be afraid of. In rare cases, large amounts of citric acid in the stomach may lead to irregularities of intestinal function. In such cases we can temporarily switch to preventative therapy dosages until our body gets used to lemon juice, and then try the healing therapy again.

In healing therapy, the following dosages are recommended:

Day 1 and 12	-	5 lemons
Day 2 and 11	-	10 lemons
Day 3 and 10	-	15 lemons
Day 4 and 9	-	20 lemons
Day 5,6,7 and 8	-	25 lemons

In total, juice squeezed from 200 lemons is consumed over 12 days. The daily amounts should be split into 3-5 dosages. Some people are terrified by the amount of juice (about one liter or quart) to be consumed on days 5, 6, 7, and 8. However, we are not afraid to drink two quarts of apple or blackcurrant juice. Lemon is just another fruit only more sour.

The therapy described above can be used for treating calcium stones. Lemon juice is one of the best remedies against them. There is an observable increase in the kidney function during the therapy. Your urine may get darker and, when allowed to stand for some time, may produce reddish sediment of uric salts. At the beginning of the therapy, one quart of urine can produce a significant amount of sediment. This means that uric acid is rapidly removed from your body thanks to the therapy. Your urine becomes amber-colored at the end of the therapy and it does not produce sediment even if allowed to stand for a long time. This means that our body does not contain excess amounts of uric acid anymore.

Lemon juice therapy is the best way to replenish vitamins in our body. We chronically suffer from vitamin deficiency, especially those who smoke (one cigarette destroys up to 25mg of vitamin C, which is a quarter of our daily recommended intake). There are still many smokers among us. Lemon juice offers wonderful benefits because citric acid is the only acid that reacts with calcium in our body, forming unique salt. As this salt is dissolved, our body receives calcium and phosphorus - elements that normalize metabolism and regenerate bone tissue.

Citric acid is also one of the products of our complex digestive process. If we supply it in the form of lemon juice, besides reducing thirst we allow our body to save energy, which can then be used for removing salty deposits from our bones, joints, muscles, and blood vessels. When citric acid reacts with amines, it forms aspartic acid that has negative charge. Natural aspartic acid formed in our body during lemon juice therapy is very valuable. Pharmaceutical formulas used in treating diseases, which were described above, contain aspartic acid in its synthetic form.

Here is some more advice on the usefulness of lemon. In cases of sore throat suck on a slice of lemon every 15 minutes - even small amounts of diluted citric acid are able to kill all germs. If you suffer from gum disease or sore gums, rinse your mouth regularly with a solution of lemon juice and warm boiled water in the morning and the evening for two weeks.

Lemon is also very effective for strengthening hair. If you have dandruff or weak hair, rub the skin on your head with a slice of lemon once a day for ten days. This will strengthen your hair and stop the formation of dandruff.

Lemon juice can also be very helpful against excessive sweating, as in the following remedy.

Remedy #6

Prepare a hot bath for your feet (2qt /2L of water with 4 teaspoons of baking soda). Soak your feet in the solution for 15-20 min. Dry the feet up and rub the toes and areas between them with a piece of lemon. During the day, you can put cotton swabs soaked in lemon juice between your toes. Repeating this routine for a few days takes care of excessive sweatiness. Additional benefit is better condition of your hands and fingernails from frequent contact with lemon juice.

If you have blisters, tape a lemon slice on top of it and leave it overnight. In the morning, the blister will be soft and easy to remove. To reduce the amount of freckles on your skin, use preventative lemon juice therapy.

In short, lemon juice is very useful against many health conditions and I encourage you to verify it on your own body.

*We are least knowledgeable about our
health, while it is the most essential
thing in our life.*

When We Suffer from Back Pains

It is hard to meet a person who would not suffer from some kind
of bone and joint pain. It makes no difference for the afflicted
person what we call the illness: rheumatism, arthritis, or osteoporosis. The label does not change the pain. I've met many
suffering people in the course of my practice. There were children, youth, and middle-aged people among them. I feel especially for the elderly because they are unhappy and helpless like
nobody else. They don't catch our attention because we don't see
them in the streets very much. In most cases, they spend a lot of
time at home alone with their pain. Most of them are already
tired of life. Sleepless nights and limited mobility result in sad
voice and tired-looking eyes. The common view is that people
are lucky if they are still alive at the age of seventy. It doesn't
bring much comfort to hear words such as, "it's hard to be old but
don't worry since you can't do anything about it." Younger people
use such phrases without thinking that, before they know it, they
will be in the same position and will be offered the same kind of
comfort.

There is a common opinion that old age comes inevitably with degenerating health. In the last several decades, the use of medications became so common that the present generation doesn't understand their proper purpose - as emergency relief for a short period in times of crises. We should take responsibility for our health, in our own hands. Medicine is focused on treating diseases but it's better for us to focus on ways to stay healthy throughout our life. The four basic principles to achieve that goal are correct breathing, physical activity, proper nutrition, and internal body hygiene. Most people have some idea about the first three but are surprised to hear about internal hygiene. We often complain about our polluted environment - dirty rivers, lead in the air, etc., but don't realize the amount of pollution inside our own body, which is reflected in our external appearance. Just look in the mirror - the spine resembles a question mark, the back is hunched, breast caved in, and the abdomen sticks forward. We feel discomfort when bending our knees, hear grinding sounds when turning the head, and don't have enough range of motion in our neck. Any kind of physical effort produces leg and back pains even in people who are still under the age of forty.

Look at what happens before holiday seasons. A lot of overweight people with swollen faces and expanded veins can be seen carrying huge boxes and bags full of sweets, pastry, meat, and deli products. From the point of view of basic health principles, what these people do is suicidal. They don't want to understand that white refined flour leads them to diabetes, milk added to pastry interferes with digestion and causes ulcers, white refined sugar impairs calcium assimilation and results in osteoporosis, while tasty deli products fill their body with uric acid and bad cholesterol that tightly "cements" blood vessels, joints and muscles. A big holiday meal stretches the stomach like a balloon and puts pressure on neighboring organs.

When all this starts causing irregular heart beat and terrible headaches, we reach for some pill to fix the problem. Frequent use of painkillers and antibiotics results in dysbacteriosis (abnormality of microflora) and a virtual hurricane of hard-to-predict biochemical anomalies in our digestive system, brought on by parasites that replace our normal healthy microflora. This means compromising our immunity and our ability to produce necessary enzymes and vitamins.

When taking an aspirin, we don't think that it might cause a hemorrhage in our stomach. It's not a big abrasion (about 3mL of blood) but the effects accumulate if we continue taking handfuls of pills to fix various problems. This is why in our degenerated gastrointestinal system, yeast and other fungi have the upper hand, which results in bloated intestines, stomach disorders, and kidney or liver stones.

The nature didn't provide us with the ability to digest antibiotics, psychotropic drugs, or painkillers. It neither gave us means to neutralize their toxic effects. These toxic compounds remain in our body for years and disturb its defensive mechanisms. If we keep taking drugs for every problem, we will inevitably fall into dependency, which affects about 60% of people with health problems. Medications cause allergic reactions in about 20% of people. I want to be understood correctly: I'm not denying the usefulness of pharmaceuticals altogether. However, every drug is a small dose of poison and should be taken only in cases of extreme crisis. Otherwise, drugs may kill us sooner than our diseases do.

Strong spirit in a strong body

In one of Canadian cities, a wheelchair-bound retired dentist attended a seminar on the therapeutic use of vegetable juices. He suffered terribly from rheumatism in all of his joints; even his jaws weren't able to chew food. Looking like a living skeleton, he had to take liquid foods through a straw. He decided to give natural therapy a try by using carrot and celery juice for nutrition and taking therapeutic hay baths. A year later he was able to open his office again and return to his normal dental practice. The only remaining sign of his past rheumatism was a slight hunch on his back.

I mentioned his case to a girl who came to me for help. Four years earlier, she suddenly started suffering from a disfiguring rheumatic disorder for no apparent reason. Her deformed fingers made her feel so uncomfortable that she stopped socializing and avoided even the closest friends. Physical pain and psychological stress resulted in apathy and depression. I had to work hard to convince her not to give up and to take initiative in the fight for her health, and eventually I was happy to see her accept the idea.

It took three years of strict dieting (practically without meat), various herbal baths, breathing exercises, drinking 1.5-2qt (1.5-2L) of juices a day, and several full body cleansing routines to achieve the desired results. Today she is completely healthy and has two beautiful daughters who are taught to respect the principles of healthy lifestyle.

I'm giving you this example to help everybody who suffers from bone and joint problems realize that they are able to help themselves. The condition will not go away in a month but given enough time under proper circumstances, our body can overcome it. This is how nature operates. It takes years for an illness to mature, and our body needs considerable time to correct the problem.

My experience shows that various problems in our skeletal system have a few main causes:

1. Internal body pollution involving lactic acid, oxalic acid, uric acid, and cholesterol
2. Physical inactivity
3. Low oxygen levels (due to eating mainly cooked food)
4. Low levels of essential micro- and macro-elements
5. Imbalance in phosphorus-calcium economy (see chapter on osteoporosis)

If we correct these deficiencies, our skeletal system problems are usually cured. I'm going to describe here, step by step, how you can achieve that. The first step to be undertaken is body detoxification, combined with a three-day fast. Freeing our body (especially the large intestine) from toxic deposits, that often poison us for years, is an essential step towards getting good results.

Body cleansing (detoxification) by fasting

During the fast, we only eat oranges and grapefruits and drink about 4 qt (4L) specially prepared juice cocktail every day. The cocktail is a mixture of 32oz (900g) of grapefruit juice, 32oz (900g) of orange juice, 7oz (200g) of lemon juice, and 2qt (2L) of distilled water, which should together give about 4L. Use only freshly squeezed juices.

Dissolve one tablespoon of Epsom salt in a glass of warm water and drink on the empty stomach in the morning. The solution acts like a magnet on impurities in our lymph. This way, toxins from all over our body are collected in the intestines and then discarded. In the process of flushing out the toxins, our body gets dehydrated. We have 4L of easily absorbable juice cocktail to compensate for the loss of water.

Dress warmly and drink 3.5oz (100g) of cocktail every 30min until the whole amount is used up. If you feel hungry, eat only oranges or grapefruits. Don't worry if you experience heavy sweating. This is normal - sweat carries away impurities from your body. Repeat the same routine on the second and third day.

Sometimes we might experience headaches, nausea, and weakness during the detoxification routine. These are temporary symptoms and, if necessary, we can alleviate them by taking a walk, massaging our ears, or chewing on a piece of lemon or orange peel. Every night before going to bed, we should drink an herbal laxative. This is necessary to help our large intestine get rid of impurities. On the forth and fifth day drink only fruit juice cocktails, for example from apples and carrots, and eat only fruits and vegetables. Grains, eggs, and fish can be added to the menu on the sixth day.

In the following 2-3 months, exclude from your diet products containing white sugar and white flour, jams, sweets, and canned goods (especially the ones containing vinegar). Limit the amounts of fried meals and fatty products, butter, cheese, eggs, meat, and fish. It's best to give up milk. You can eat up to 50g a day of white cottage cheese (made from full milk) and drink up to one glass of sour milk. The basis of our diet should be grains, salads, fruits, vegetables, and their freshly squeezed juices. Using proper combinations of food products is very important. (Table 2, page 52)

I'm going to present here just the general guidelines for correctly combining foods. We have to make sure that our body is supplied all the nutrition it needs and doesn't suffer deficiency or excess of any essential substances. All components of a meal should be digested in roughly the same amount of time. This eliminates the possibility of undigested chunks of food getting into our intestines and causing unhealthy consequences. The principles of correctly combining food products are based on millennia-old experience and are a valuable gift from our ancestors. They give wonderful results. The basic idea is not combining certain types of food products at the same meal.

For example, digestion time for proteins is 2-4 hours, while for carbohydrates 20-40 minutes. The usual mass of carbohydrates we eat is much bigger than the mass of proteins. Undigested protein chunks can get to duodenum together with the large mass of carbohydrates, and this must be prevented.

Proteins are digested by acid-active enzymes while the digestion of carbohydrates requires alkaline-active enzymes. They neutralize each other in the stomach and additional amounts of acid-active enzymes have to be secreted. If our stomach contains a mixture of carbohydrates and proteins (as in a typical meal), the amount of acid-active enzyme needed to digest, for example, 3.5oz (100g) of meat is 20-25 times higher than normal. At the same time carbohydrates and other components of the meal remain undigested.

All food products are commonly divided into four groups:

1. Proteins - meat, fish, eggs, beans, nuts, etc.
2. Carbohydrates - bread, candy, potatoes, honey, sugar, etc.
3. Fats - butter, oil, grease, etc.
4. Fruits and vegetables, fruit juices

The principles of combining these food groups are described below.

Table 2: Combining food products

PROTEIN RICH FOODSM	FATS AND "LIVE" PRODUCTS	CARBOHYDRATE FOODS
eat and meat soups, fish, eggs, egg-plant, beans, Windsor beans, nuts, sunflower seeds, plain yogurt, kefir, cottage cheese, buttermilk, sour milk	Grease, butter, vegetable oil, fruits (raw or dried), vegetables (raw or dried, except potatoes), fruit and vegetable juices.	Breads and other flour based prod-ucts, grains, pota-toes, sugar, honey, products contain-ing sugar, pasta, jams, candies
	It is better to always consume milk, dry wine, melon and banana separately from other products	
Can be combined		Can be combined

Foods in the middle column can be combined with either protein foods in the first or carbohydrate foods in the third column, but foods in the first and the third columns should never be combined.

These rules for combining foods may be hard to accept for some people, because they are used to eating meat with bread, buns, potatoes, or rice. However in the end, the most impor-tant consideration is our health.

In the annex, p. 215-222 I give a few examples of healthy meals that are suitable both for healthy people and those encountering health problems.

I suggest eating two full meals a day - the first between 8 and 9 a.m. and the second between 5 and 8 p.m. We can eat fruits and vegetables as snacks between meals. For drinking use freshly squeezed fruit or vegetable juices and good quality water. Best of all, drink green tea or herbal tea (chamomile, nettle, melissa, etc.)

Chew your food thoroughly, at least 30 times for each bite. Don't drink while you eat your solid food. Your meals should be arranged in the following manner:

1. Juice, tea or mineral water
2. Salad
3. Main course (carbohydrates in the morning and proteins in the evening)

For healthy people, carrot and beat juice cocktail (4:1 ratio) is very useful to drink as a preventative measure against health problems. There are not very many people who are completely healthy and optimal juice combinations are different for different cases. Since we've been talking about skeletal system problems, I'm going to mention a few juice cocktails that strengthen our bones. Drink your juice cocktails 2-3 times a day, 15-20min before or 1-1.5hr after meals. They should be helpful in cases of bone, muscle and spine problems, as well as joint inflammations, osteoporosis, tooth decay, podagra, rheumatism, and gum disease. The amounts of juices below are intended for a single drink.

1. Carrot 9oz (250g)
2. Carrot 8oz (230g) + lettuce 5oz (140g) + spinach 3oz (85g)

3. Carrot 10oz (280g) + spinach 6oz (170g)
4. Carrot 8oz (230g) + celery 115g + parsley root 2.1oz(60g) + spinach 3oz (85g)
5. Carrot 8oz (230g) + beet 3oz (85g) + cucumber 3oz (85g)
6. Carrot 320g + beet 3oz (85g) + coconut 2.1oz (60g)
5. Spinach 7oz (200g)
6. Carrot 8oz (230g) + celery 5oz (140g) + parsley root 2.1oz (60g)
7. Lemon 7oz (200g)

It's best to prepare vegetable juice cocktails directly before drinking, in any case not longer than 8-10 hours earlier if we can store them refrigerated in the temperature 32-46F (0-8C). The next component of our meal should be salads. Make sure they are tasty, and preferably made from locally grown vegetables in their natural vegetation season. The more different colors we have in our salads the healthier they are (see annex p. 215-222).

It's not aging that degenerates our spine

Life in our civilized society doesn't require much physical effort. Physical inactivity and incorrect nutrition cause our spine to become inflexible. Damaged vertebrae and discs result in spine's deformation. As a matter, of course, we blame aging for these problems. In reality, aging as such doesn't have anything to do with them. Take a close look at the way many children move, with their hunched backs and stiff legs. If they continue this way, the degenerative changes build up, but it doesn't mean that aging as such is to be blamed for it.

I've met many people who were over a hundred years old and still had a strong and healthy spine, were able to work, and were usually in good spirits. People complain about their spine problems, ignoring their own negligence as the cause. I once had the pleasure to watch the 80th birthday performance of Mahmud Isymbayev, a well-known dancer. Slim and youthful in appearance, dynamic and energetic in his performance, he danced almost continuously for 1.5 hours. When he bowed to the audience at the end, he almost reached the floor with his forehead. This proves that our spine's shape doesn't depend on the age but on proper nutrition and adequate amount of physical activity.

I'd like to mention three cases of seemingly unrelated health problems from my practice. After closer examination they all turned out to originate from the same source and proved a close relation between our general health and the condition of our spine.

Case Number 1

A couple was seeking help for their 15 year-old daughter who found herself in a tragic predicament. For no obvious reason, the left side of her face became disfigured, her left eye couldn't close and she wasn't able to raise the eyebrow. She had been treated with injections and physiotherapy for a month without any results. For the young girl, such plainly visible disfiguration was of course a psychological trauma. I first paid attention to the way she walked - the movements were very stiff. Further examination involved raising and lowering her arms, sitting down, standing up, and finally taking shoes off and trying to keep balance on one foot. She could do it only for several seconds.

Tibetan monks use this method of examination whenever they suspect misalignment of lumbar vertebrae, especially the first vertebra. It controls all vertical movements of our body: raising and lowering of arms, opening and closing of eyes, as well as standing up. Difficulties with any of these movements indicate fatigue and hardening of the first vertebra.

Modern diagnostic methods aren't able to detect those changes. There are techniques to correct such condition. I "unblocked" the vertebra and prescribed a set of exercises that she was able to do on her own in order to correct spinal misalignment and regain all functions controlled by the first vertebra. I saw her several times a month to check the progress.

It took two months for everything to go back to normal. Her facial muscles started working properly and the eye could close. Her doctor was amazed at the recovery because he couldn't get any significant results with other patients suffering from the same condition.

Coincidentally, one of the doctors in the same clinic suffered from the same neurological problem. He was even more puzzled when he found out that medication prescribed the girl by his colleague was the same he was taking without any results. This is a good illustration of what Hippocrates meant when he said, "Every illness has its cause that cannot be removed by taking medications."

Case Number 2

Ancient medicine has in its arsenal hundreds of ways to diagnose by external symptoms. Facial wrinkles, the color and shape of ears, shape of fingernails, wearing out of shoes, etc., can tell the story of internal diseases. The Chinese can diagnose over 300 ailments by examining the pulse, and Tibetan lamas can tell 150 diseases based on individual body smell.

I have an unconscious habit of watching for certain external signs and analyzing the health level in people I meet. Sometimes when we watch TV, my wife asks me about the health of politicians or performers appearing on the screen. Once I told her that her favorite singer's limping is caused by a degenerated second lumbar vertebra. She didn't believe me because she knew that his limping was attributed to injury suffered in an accident. I still argued that spine-aligning therapy could take care of the problem. A few months later the singer contacted me asking for an appointment. As it turned out, he had gotten one of my books as a birthday gift and got interested in seeking some help for his health problems. During the consultation, he told me about his accident and about progressive walking difficulties. His doctors suggested hip surgery, but he wanted to consider alternative treatments. I asked him to try a few test exercises designed to examine the condition of the second lumbar vertebra, which proved my earlier diagnosis. Then I explained that the second lumbar vertebra is responsible for maintaining body balance in left-right motions, which influences the way we walk. Limping is in most cases an indication of a dislocated second lumbar vertebra. I finally convinced him by helping him to put his spine in order. He never had to go through a surgery and now he walks normally without using his cane. He started paying attention to his health. I hope he will keep it up to become even more healthy and energetic.

In my other book ("Can We Live 150 Years?"), I said more about spine maintenance. I would only like to add here that exercising our spine is necessary to keep cartilaginous discs in good shape, which prevents their flattening and painful friction between our vertebrae.

When calcium level in the discs goes down, our spine loses its shock-absorbing qualities. Friction and pressure between vertebrae cause pinching of nerves that branch out of our spinal cord and exit through spaces between vertebrae. Luckily, special exercises can quickly regenerate cartilaginous discs. This is possible at any age, provided proper nutrition and exercising routine. Even if you are advanced in years, you can regenerate your discs and maintain your whole spine as healthy as young people.

Case Number 3

A 34-year-old man came to me for consultation. He had problems with erection and urination. A treatment prescribed by his urologist had resulted in some improvement but failed to bring back full sexual performance. On top of that, he encountered frequent constipation.

In cases of erection problems, the likely "culprit" is usually the third lumbar vertebra. Stiffness in both the second and the third vertebrae results in constipation, erection problems, and finally prostate gland inflammation. Since many men have to deal with those serious and troublesome conditions that are related, I'll try to explain their common origin.

The anatomy of male urogenital system is well-known. Some of its components are urethra coming out of the bladder, prostate gland, seminal vesicles, and testes. Prostate gland consists of muscle tissue and hormone-producing tissue. The testes produce sperm and seminal vesicles secrete mucous that allows sperm to survive. All these three elements join to form semen and are entered together into urethra. When the intestine expands as it fills with hardened deposits (due to eating meat and white flour products, sedentary lifestyle, etc.), the prostate gland gets squeezed by the expanding intestine. As a result, it develops more muscle tissue and produces smaller amounts of hormones, which follows by lower mucus production and "drying up" of seminal vesicles. The pressure on the prostate gland is also transferred to urethra, which causes urination difficulties. The best course of action is taking four steps:

1. Cleaning up the large intestine (p. 141)
2. Changing nutritional habits (Table 2, p. 52)
3. Drinking a lot of vegetable juices (e.g. lemon therapy p. 40-42; carrot 10oz (280g) + beets 3.2oz (90g) + cucumber 3.2oz (90g) - twice a day; carrot 9oz (250g) - twice a day)
4. Regenerating your vertebrae by exercising (p. 61-63)

This method should take care of urination problems in 15-20 days, cure prostate inflammation soon after, and return everything to full functionality in 5-6 months without the need for any surgery.

The lumbar section of our spine has five vertebrae (six in rare cases). We already know the consequences of stiffness and fatigue in the first three. What are the other two vertebra involved in? The fourth vertebra deals with body movements when sitting down and determines moments of sexual arousal. Degeneration of this vertebra can cause pain while sitting down, abnormal weight, lack of sexual excitement, and uterus disorders. The fifth vertebra directs back-and-forth motions, for example while walking, working, or during the sexual act. It also deals with respiratory functions and skin condition.

This was a general description of the relation between the condition of our lumbar spine and certain motor functions. You can perform a test consisting of leaning sideways, backwards and forwards, sitting down, and standing up. If you have difficulty performing these movements and feel pressure in the lumbar area, your lumbar vertebrae are stiff and dysfunctional, and that negatively influences many aspects of your health.

Due to inactive lifestyle, there are few people whose lumbar spine is completely healthy. Pains in the lumbar area are usually treated with baths, massage, rub-on medications, or injections of B group vitamins. These methods give only temporary relief because they only fight symptoms. If the true cause is not removed, the condition will deteriorate in the long run.

Lumbar vertebrae are closely related with our hips. Bones and joints of our pelvic area are responsible for all motor functions in our body. Our hips are structurally a very important part of our body. They can be compared to the foundation of a house or the root system of a tree because of the way they support the upper body. Our pelvis participates in six types of motion: up, down, forward, backward, opening, and closing. Difficulties in performing any of these movements are an indication of deformations. The center of the pelvis may be shifted up or down and the spine may be slightly misaligned. If the deformations grow, vertebrae start pinching nerves that branch out of the spinal cord. We start experiencing pain in the internal organs those nerves are connected to. The bigger the deformations are the more serious consequences we suffer.

The effects of deformation can spread upwards (dizziness, headaches, ringing in the ears) or downwards (pains in the knees, feet, or heels). Spine deformations are, to some degree, the result of our body's self-balancing mechanism. If you tried to tilt your head back and walk that way for a few minutes, you'll start swaying to the sides, feel psychological discomfort, fear, and something strange happening with your brain.

Our self-balancing mechanism intended to keep the brains position in a safe range involves the property of parallelism built into our eyes. The spine changes its alignment because of that mechanism. You can sometimes notice people with imperfect jaw or shoulder symmetry, or with a deformed chest cage. Many of these deformities are caused by improper alignment in the pelvic section. This is why eastern medicine pays so much attention to that area.

A healthy spine is the foundation of good health.

Nutrition, hygiene, psychological factors, breathing, and aerobic or aquatic exercises are all important, but without a healthy spine they all will not make you feel really healthy. What can we do to maintain it in a really good shape?

1. Sleep on a firm mattress or on the floor (see "Can We Live 150 Years?" page 43)
2. Use a small firm pillow or a rolled-up towel under your neck
3. Eat only healthy food types and drink a lot of juices
4. Cleanse your skeletal system (Remedies# 3, 5, 21)
5. Take therapeutic baths
6. Exercise daily

You can perform your favorite set of exercises or use one of the sets suggested below. They help in aligning your vertebrae and removing tension from your skeletal system. Try one of them before you go on reading. Remember it and perform twice a day at your convenience (at home, work, gas station, etc.) Most people's spines resemble old rusty mechanisms because they spend 80% of their time in a bent, sitting, or lying position. **If you dedicate some time to your spine's condition, the reward will be a significant improvement in your health.**

Exercise set number 1

Exercise #1
Lying on your back, your arms alongside the body, palms down, pull up your knees trying to reach the forehead then

stretch them again. Repeat the exercise 10 times.

Exercise #2
Stand up, bend forward and try to reach the floor with your fingers (palms, if you can). Bow your head back and forth, following the movements of your torso. Stand straight, your legs slightly apart, and close your fists.

Exercise #3
Rotate your both arms 10 times forward and 10 times back.

Exercise #4
Tilt sideways left and right, sliding your hands alongside your body until you reach the knee. Turn your head left and right at the same time.

Exercise #5
With your feet slightly apart, raise your right hand and reach over to the left shoulder blade, lower your hand, then raise the left hand and reach over to the right shoulder blade. Repeat 10 times.

Exercise #6
With your feet slightly apart, raise your both hands and rotate your torso clockwise 10 times and counterclockwise 10 times.

Exercise #7
With your feet slightly apart and your torso in a vertical position, try to reach your chest with your left and then with your with right knee. Repeat 10 times.

Exercise #8

Holding on to the back of a chair, do at least 10 sit-down exercises.

Try to repeat each exercise 10 times at first and gradually increase the number of repetitions to 20-40.

It can emanate from your mind

Pains in the back and lumbar area not always originate from vertebra dislocation. The source can sometimes be psychological problems. People's posture can tell you more about the spirits they are in. Those who are confident and relaxed tend to keep a straight posture and usually look up. Distressed, disturbed, or saddened people lower their heads and recoil their shoulders. It can be explained the following way: anger, irritation, sadness, or any kind of psychological discomfort trigger tension, contraction, and stiffness of our spinal muscles. That in turn puts pressure on neural networks running through the muscles and causes the sensation of pain.

People who are fearful and passive in dealing with stressful situations, make decisions slowly and indecisively, and tend to isolate themselves, are bound to suffer from frequent back pains. If this sounds like some of your personality traits, it's likely that there is a psychological factor in your back troubles. According to statistics, it is a contributing component in every second case. There are some helpful techniques helping to reduce tensions in your body. By applying these uncomplicated techniques of regulating your mood you can regain the natural harmony of your body and mind. In 10-20 minutes, you can achieve full relaxation and completely release tension from your muscles. You can exercise with a quiet relaxing music in the background if you like.

Exercise #9

Lower and relax your arms. Shake them gently as if you tried to shake off droplets of water. Do the same with your feet. Raise your hands as if you tried to reach the sun. Imagine that your body becomes heavy and behaves like a long-stemmed water lily. Start leaning towards the floor. Close your eyes and try to feel your body weight more and more. Lie on your back and spread your arms and legs. Concentrate on the tips of your toes and think how heavy and inert they are. The feeling of heaviness takes over your feet, legs, hips, torso, arms, and fingers, as if your body were filled with some heavy matter. Your chin goes down towards your chest. Imagine that something is stretching all your facial muscles in all directions. Try to believe you are heavy enough to sink into the ground. Relax your breath, inhaling and exhaling as slowly as possible. Now picture a light white cloud moving across the sky. Imagine you are becoming that cloud and your body is very light and calm. You glide effortlessly in the sky over fields, woods, and waters. Try to smell flowers, trees, or the sea. Remain in this relaxed state as long as you want.

You can picture your fingers become tube-like and let tensions, distress, and fatigue out of your body. When you feel that all tension is gone, slowly make your entire body feel firm again. Put your arms over your head and stretch your entire body. Slowly roll over on your right side, flex and stretch like babies waking up from their sleep, then do it again lying on your left side. Sit up slowly, stretch again, and open your eyes. Stand up slowly and return to your normal activities. Your muscles should feel rested, your mood balanced, and your spirit rejuvenated.

For those who are usually short of time, I suggest the following set of exercises:

Exercise set number 2

These exercises are easy to do, even for ill people. They wonderfully relax and remove fatigue caused by long hours of sitting work, when our head feels heavy and all our muscles are tense. The exercises can be done anywhere - at work, at a bus stop, or even while on the phone.

Exercise #1 - Vibro-massage
  Rise on your toes to have your heels 1-2 cm above the floor, then drop back on your heels with the entire body weight. Don't hurry - do it about every second for a total of sixty times. Those involved in long sitting work should do this exercise 3-5 times a day. It's a good preventative exercise against varicose veins and heart disorders.

Exercises that utilize urinary and anal sphincter mechanisms (muscles that hold back urination and defecation) are unique in their simplicity and extraordinary in their effectiveness. Their secret was preserved for a long time by yoga masters. They promote muscle relaxation, improve blood circulation, and prevent reproductive system disorders in men and women. They can be done anywhere without even being noticed.

Exercise #2 - Front lock (kegel exercises)
  It is done by contracting the urinary sphincter muscle. We do it automatically when we have to hold before we can get

to the restroom or when we complete urinating. You do it consciously when you want to pause urinating. The exercise consists of doing the same kind of muscle contraction 5-10 times. Perform this exercise 3-5 times a day.

Exercise #3 - Anal lock
This exercise is done by repeated contraction the anal sphincter muscle, as if you wanted to stop a stool (3-5 times daily).

Exercise #4 - Double lock
Perform 10 simultaneous contractions of both sphincters (best on exhaling). It has a double effect. Perform once a day.

Many people walk with their back bowed, as if they were burdened with a heavy load all their life. If you try to keep your head raised, your back straight, and your eyes joyfully bright, many of your health problems will disappear. Here are some exercises that can help you maintain happy and cheerful appearance.

Exercise #5
Lean against the wall with your heals, buttocks, and head for 3-5 minutes. Pull in your stomach, look straight ahead and think that nobody in the world is as happy and good-looking as you are. This should fill your muscles with a warm sensation and bring brightness to your eyes. Try to always keep that feeling in your mind.

The following exercise is for those who spend a lot of time on their feet or in a sitting position. It is designed to quickly remove tension from all muscles.

Exercise #6
Stand on one leg and bend the other knee until you reach your buttock with the heel. Support the knee with your hand and remain so for 1-2 minutes, then do the same with the other leg.

Joint, bone, and muscle pains

So far, I explained a few causes of pains and methods of prevention. If you've been suffering from old persistent aches and pains in your joints, bones, and muscles, try some of the following remedies.

Remedy #7 (for strong pains, as in nerve inflammations)
Tape horseradish leaves on the painful area for a few days (until the pain stops). You can use fresh leaves every day.

Remedy #8 (for eliminating pains caused by deposits of salts)
Boil some rye flour and blend with an equal amount of boiled potatoes to get a uniform mass. Rub some vegetable oil on the affected spot and massage it well. Form a loaf out of the blended mass. Put some turpentine on the affected area and the loaf on top of it. Cover yourself with a warm blanket and remain so as long as possible (e.g. overnight).

Remedy #9 (for eliminating pains caused by deposits of salts)
Grind 3 lemons (complete - with the peel) and 5.3oz (150g) of peeled garlic; mix them, and pour 0.5qt (0.5L) of boiled water on the mixture. Let it stand for 24 hours, then strain it, squeeze all juice from the grinds and pour it into a glass jar with a tight lid. Take 1.8oz (50g) a day before breakfast.

Remedy #10 (against joint pains)
Blend 2 glasses of radish juice with 1 glass of honey, 0.5 glass of vodka, and a teaspoon of salt. Rub on the affected spots.

Remedy #11
Mix 1.5 cup of black radish juice with 1 cup of honey, (150mL) of vodka (40% proof or stronger) and 1 tablespoon of salt. Take 1 tablespoon before bedtime. Store refrigerated.

Remedy #12
Grind enough parsley (complete - with root and green) to get one cup of grinds. Put it in a pot, pour 2 cups of boiling water on it, cover with a towel, and leave overnight. Strain the mixture in the morning and squeeze one average-sized lemon into the juice. Drink 1/3 of a cup twice a day after meals for 2 days; make a three-day interval, and continue that way until the pain stops.

Remedy #13
Ingredients: 0.5 quart (0.5L) of vodka (40% proof or stronger), 5 pods of hot pepper 2.5-3 inches (6-8cm) long.
Preparation: Chop the pepper pods finely, put in a jar, pour spirit over it, cover with a lid, and let it stand in a dark place for a week.
Usage: Soak a piece of cotton cloth in the formula and cover the affected area for 3-4 hours. Even the most persistent pains should disappear after 7-10 sessions.

Remedy #14
Ingredients: 1.8oz (50g) of camphor, 1.8oz (50g) of powdered mustard seed, 0.35oz (10g) of vodka (40% proof or

up), 3.5oz (100g) of raw egg white.

Preparation: Pour spirit in a jar, add camphor, and let it dissolve. Add and dissolve mustard seed powder, add egg white, and stir to form a thick pulp. Keep refrigerated and warm up slightly before each use.

Usage: Rub on the effected muscle and joint areas before bedtime. Do not rub in completely - let it leave a film on your skin for 20 minutes and then wash the excess off with a piece of cotton cloth soaked in warm water.

Remedy #15 (against rheumatism)
Chop finely a sunflower head and put in a 1qt (1L) jar together with 1.8oz (50g) of soap flakes. Pour 0.5qt (500mL) of vodka on it, stir well, put a tight lid on it, and let it stand in sunlight for 8-9 days. Then stir again, strain, squeeze all liquid from the pulp, and pour the liquid into a glass jar with a tight lid. Rub on affected areas.

Remedy #16 (against rheumatism)
Grate and squeeze enough turnip to get one and a half cups of juice. Add one cup of honey, half a cup of vodka, and a tablespoon of salt. Mix well, put in a jar with a tight lid, and store in a cool place. Use it as a rub.

Remedy #17 (against osteoporosis)
Pour 0.5qt (0.5L) of boiling water on two tablespoons of rice and let it stand overnight. Strain the water out in the morning and cook the rice. Eat on an empty stomach, without salt, two hours before a meal, every day for a total of forty days. Repeat the therapy after a few months' interval.

Remedy #18 (against rheumatism and arthritis)
Chop up four lemons, mix with 3 cups of water, and boil

together until there is only about 1 cup of mixture remaining. Let it cool down and strain it. Mix it with 1 cup of honey and juice from 1 lemon. Keep in a glass jar with a lid. Take 1 tablespoon before going to bed.

Remedy #19 (against rheumatism and arthritis)
Mix 7oz (200g) of ground horseradish with 7oz (200g) of rye flour and 2 tablespoons of turpentine. Keep in a glass jar with a lid. Form the pulp into a loaf, put it on the affected area, and wrap a towel around it. Keep it for 5-8 hours (best overnight).

Remedy #20 (against rheumatism and arthritis)
Add 1.8oz (50g) of finely chopped birch buds to 0.5qt (0.5L) of vodka. Let it stand 10 days in a dark place. Strain and squeeze the liquid out, put in a bottle, and close tightly. Take 1 teaspoon 3 times a day with some water.

Remedy #21 (cleansing your bones and joints)
One stage of the therapy takes three consecutive days and uses about 0.5oz (15g) of bay leaves.

Day 1 - Break up 0.18oz (5g) of bay leaves, put in 10 fl oz (300 mL) of boiling water, and boil slowly for 5 minutes. Pour into a thermos and put aside for 5 hours to settle. Strain it into another container and drink in small sips every 15-20 minutes over 12 hours.
Note: Never drink the entire extract at one time - this could cause a hemorrhage.

Day 2 and 3 - Continue as on the first day.

During the therapy eliminate meat, eggs, cheese, cottage cheese, etc. from your menu.

As salts and sand are excreted during the therapy, your urine's color may change to any from green to light red. This is a normal phenomenon. It is a two-stage therapy with a seven-day interval and it should be used once a year. The best time to undergo this therapy is the summer-fall season.

The best benefit a book can bring is not only revealing the truth but also inspiring insight.

No Such Thing as Bad Weather

Researches calculated that one person out of three reacts to sudden weather changes. For unknown reasons women suffer twice as much as men. The usual symptoms are fatigue, nausea, heavy sweating, anxiety, and migraine pains. In reality the weather itself doesn't cause any harm, only helps reveal our health deficiencies. If all our metabolic processes are very regular, our circulatory system is used to rapid expansion and contraction of blood vessels, our nerves are "made of steel", and our thinking is dominated by positive ideas, then weather changes cannot do us any harm. Here is a quick test determining your sensitivity to weather changes.

1. Do you feel restless?
2. Do you experience excessive sweating in the morning?
3. Do you feel tired in the morning and have difficulty getting up?
4. Do you feel better when it gets cooler?
5. Do you feel approaching weather changes?

If you answered "yes" to only one question, you are not sensitive to weather changes. Two positive answers are no cause to panic, but they mean you should undertake some steps to prevent "weather sensitivity." Four positive answers mean high sensitivity and a necessity for immediate action.

To develop tolerance to weather changes, you need to work on the hardiness of your nervous system and blood vessels. Regular use of the following routines helps activate your defense mechanisms and make the weather your ally.

Relaxing hand massage

This massage routine relaxes the nervous system, enhances circulation, improves vision, and slows the aging processes.

Remedy #22

Sit down comfortably, relax your muscles (especially facial muscles), and close your eyes. Imagine some natural setting e.g. ocean, forest, or mountains. Take deep breaths through the nose and exhale slowly through the mouth with your lips rounded. When you feel relaxed, start massaging the little finger of your left hand using the thumb and index finger of your right hand. The motion should imitate screwing a bolt in. Go on massaging the other fingers and the thumb and then do the same with the other hand. Each finger and thumb should be massaged for about one minute.

Alternate hot and cold showers

It turns out that by simply applying cold and hot water we can get unexpectedly good results in fighting many diseases. The importance of the alternate use of cold and heat lies in the fact that heat stimulates the surface areas of our body and increases blood supply to the skin while cold stimulates blood circulation in our internal organs. By doing so, the alternate action of cold and heat in water therapy becomes a miraculous cure for many diseases because it regulates blood circulation, strengthens our muscles and heart, and improves our immune system.

Adjust the water temperature to make it comfortable and pleasant for 40 seconds. Use the cold-water knob to decrease the temperature (within the comfort zone) for 20 seconds, and then increase it again using the same knob. Follow the pattern: 40 seconds - warm, 20 seconds - cold. Repeat for 3-5 minutes, depending on how you feel.

When in the shower, imagine that muscle tension and nervous stress are being rinsed off your body. Get used to regular alternate hot and cold showers in the morning and evening, and whenever you feel tired, annoyed, or weak. No weather changes will affect you anymore.

Alternate cold and warm massage

Alternate cold and warm massage decreases our body's sensitivity to cold and heat and refreshes our nervous system. It is particularly advisable for elderly people because it decreases their proneness to fatigue and sweating, the sensitivity of their muscles and joints, and their reaction to weather changes. The effects are even better if extracts of chamomile, sage, or other medicinal herbs are added to water used in the massage. This provides a double benefit for wilted skin - the benefits of the massage and of the vitamins contained in the extracts.

Remedy #23

Soak a small towel in cold water, wring it out and massage one of your arms. The same routine should be repeated for the other arm, the chest, back, and legs. The total time for the entire body should be 3-5 minutes. It is best to use this therapy every morning after an alternate cold and hot shower. Let your skin dry off a little for about two minutes before you use a towel.

Healing water

Each organism begins its life in water; a human fetus is no exception. Kneip, a German physician, in his book "Wasser Erleben und Erfahren" wrote: "Each contact with water means an additional minute in our life". Recent scientific research proves that our body can most easily rebuilt its natural electric potential with the help of water. It is no coincidence that many cultures' customs include rituals such as offering water to travelers or baptizing babies with water. Both Hippocrates in ancient Greece and Avicenna, Persian physician and philosopher in medieval times, extensively used water therapy by applying alternately cold and hot water and then massaging a patient's body. This kind of therapy improves blood circulation and metabolism, helps to eliminate excess mucus out of the body, and consequently causes a speedy healing process. **People are often ready to travel hundreds of miles looking for a mi-**

raculous cure but they do not realize that better results can be achieved using regular water flowing out of their tap. Seneca, a great philosopher, was right when he remarked that the essence of things is in their simplicity.

People who don't believe in therapeutic properties of water should remember that life is always associated with the presence of water. As soon as they start using water remedies, they will be on the way to freedom from many health problems.

Therapeutic breathing exercises

Many people experience headaches, nausea, and anxiety whenever a barometric high is approaching. This is especially true for people with low blood pressure. If we frequently suffer from such symptoms, we should try to understand their causes and learn some useful remedies.

As a warm front approaches, our body produces higher amounts of adrenaline, the heart rate increases, and we become anxious. At the same time, our blood vessels expand and there is a sensation of air shortage. All these symptoms are directly or indirectly related to low oxygen levels in our body. Other symptoms include increased anxiety, insomnia or sleepiness, and depression. In addition to remedies mentioned above, performing the following breathing exercises once a day can help the situation.

Remedy #24 (helpful against anxiety, insomnia, and headaches)
Put a straw in your mouth, sit straight with your head raised, inhale through your nose and exhale through the straw. Do it in a relaxed and regular manner for 3-5 minutes. The straw is there to slow down your exhaling, which helps in

completely removing harmful substances from your lungs. This is a very simple but effective way to increase oxygen level in your blood

Here is one more breathing exercise:

Remedy #25 (normalizes heart beat, helps in overcoming panic attacks, releases the   feeling of heaviness in the heart area, increases circulation)

Breathe only through your nose. Exhale slowly and completely and then take a rapid short breath. Try to do your best to imitate a sigh. This is helpful in releasing muscle and nervous system tensions brought by trauma or stressful situations. Repeat the exercise at least 20 times.

Sniffing valerian drops

Most of us know that stimulating the nasal partition with ammonia smell brings immediate result in cases of fainting or alcohol poisoning. Our nasal partition is responsible for the physiological balance of all our bodily organs. By stimulating it with various smells, we can directly and effectively influence the function of many organs and systems. Sniffing valerian drops helps reduce blood pressure, improves sleep, quiets the nervous system, and enhances immunity. The therapy should be done daily before going to bed, for 3-4 months. There are usually noticeable effects after the first month in the form of general rejuvenation and increased strength. It's not uncommon for graying hair to darken again during this therapy.

Remedy #26

Use only pure alcohol-based valerian drops that don't contain any other heart medication. Inhaling should be slow and deep. Close one nostril with your finger, hold valerian drops close to the other nostril, inhale and exhale slowly 3 to 5 times, and then do the same with the other nostril.

This therapy is very helpful in insomnia cases. When you wake up too soon, repeat the routine. If your head doesn't feel quite clear in the morning, increase the number of inhalations the next evening, until you arrive at your own optimal number.

Help your heart

People with heart problems are most sensitive to weather changes. It's a serious mistake for them to lie in bed when they don't feel well. This puts on their heart the whole burden of pumping blood through inefficient blood vessels.

There are about 600 muscles in human body. Blood vessels form a network around each muscle, and all muscle movements help in moving blood along. This means we have 600 additional small "hearts" we can utilize by keeping our body active. The more muscles are engaged the better for our heart, the rest of circulatory system, and our health in general. Undoubtedly the best kind of exercise that helps our heart and decreases sensitivity to weather changes is outdoor walking. It involves most of our muscles; even internal organs react to our steps (put you hands on your belt area while walking to feel muscle movements).

Walk away from the risk of heart attack. Regular fast walks help reduce the risk of heart attack and stroke by 40%. This was a conclusion from an American study involving 85 thousand women.

Dr. G. Monson in a Boston women's clinic studied for eight years the health condition of nurses aged 40-65. He concluded that half of them maintained good health thanks to their habitual energetic way of walking. Three hours' worth of brisk walk every week cuts in half the risk of heart attack by normalizing blood pressure, reducing cholesterol level, and keeping weight under control. It also lowers the probability of diabetes.

This was known already in ancient Greece. For example, Aristotle maintained that nothing is as detrimental to our health as long physical inactivity. It took us thousands of years to finally come to the same conclusions.

Everybody benefits from physical exercise, young and old alike. Ill people need exercise much more than those who are healthy. Those with heart and circulatory disorders can make themselves less sensitive to barometric pressure changes, magnetic storms, solar storms, and the like. Exercising promotes health. Do whatever you are able to do - run, walk, or even crawl - as long as it keeps you from too much lying and sitting down.

All businessmen and businesswomen would probably argue that it is easy for me to give such advice from a country retreat or a quiet office, while they have to contend with daily stress and worries, can afford only three to five hours of sleep, and hardly have time to swallow a pill when something goes wrong with their health.

In reply I would inform them that I think about the content of my future books while I take morning power walks (6-7.5 miles /10-12km) that allow me to maintain a good shape, strong heart, and excellent memory. I have had difficult times in my life when I was not able to walk, not even get out of bed for two years because of spinal injury. However, my love for life and the desire to be healthy allowed me to heal my spine and start helping others in dealing with similar problems.

Following is a set of exercises that played an important role in my rehabilitation. It can be performed first thing in the morning, while you are still in bed. If used regularly, it can put your nervous system in order, improve the function of the endocrine glands, enhance your stamina, and increase your hardiness in dealing with stress. I suggest that you pause your reading and try these exercises now.

Exercise set number 3

Exercise #1
Put your thumbs behind the ears and the other fingers against the ears. Massage your ears performing up and down movements of your index fingers.

Exercise #2
Put your right hand against the forehead to have the little finger on the left eyebrow. Then put your left hand on top of the right with the little finger against the right eyebrow. Rub your forehead with left and right movements of both hands (30 times), keeping your little fingers on the eyebrows.

Exercise #3
Close your eyes, put your thumbs against the eyelids, and massage your eyes with circular motion (15 times clockwise and 15 times counterclockwise).

Exercise #4
Put your right hand on the abdomen, cover it and press with your left hand, and massage your abdomen using circular motion 30 times clockwise. Switch your hands and massage 30 times counterclockwise.

81

Exercise #5

Pull in your stomach as much as possible, and then expand it like a balloon. Repeat 30 times.

Exercise #6

Put hands on your neck and interlock your fingers; massage the neck 30 times horizontally and 30 times vertically

There is much talk about life "in the fast lane" causing heart attacks. We use terms such as "stress" or "daily tensions" to explain higher mortality rates due to heart attacks. I would not make the connection between nervous tension and heart attacks, particularly among younger population. The real cause is simpler than that. The body is poisoned internally due to unhealthy lifestyle. Insoluble calcium salts and bad cholesterol deposits damage our blood vessels. In addition, blood is thick and acidic, which inevitably causes clots. This means that all people who don't start taking care of their heart early enough can, sooner or later, expect a heart attack.

I have known many people who did not discriminate in their food and drink choices, did not put any limits on the amounts they consumed, and could spend entire nights in front of computer screens in their offices filled with tobacco smoke and strong coffee aroma. They never had time for a walk and their phone was ringing almost 24 hours a day. They often believed to be in good shape because they were not suffering from any pains. Even when they fell down with a heart attack, they still refused to blame their lifestyle for it. According to them, the cause was work-related stress and daily worries.

As we know from history, human beings have always lived under stress. We cannot even imagine the stress our distant ancestors must have experienced when they were in danger of being attacked by a wild animal at any moment. They had very

them, add 2.2lb (1kg) of honey to the juice and mix well. Peel and grind 10 big heads of garlic, put the grinds in a jar and blend with lemon juice and honey. Wrap the jar in a dark towel and let it stand in the refrigerator for 7 days. After that period, stir the mixture well and take 1 teaspoon 3-4 times a day. The amount should last you about 2 months. Take a four-month interval, then prepare the mixture again the same way and repeat the therapy. If you do this regularly, you won't have to worry about the condition of your blood vessels.

Remedy #28
Mix 1 glassful of Italian dill seeds with 2 tablespoons of ground valerian roots and 2 cups of honey. Put the mixture into a 2qt (2L) thermos and fill it with boiling water. Leave it stand for 24 hours, then strain it into a jar and store on the lowest shelf in your refrigerator. Take 1 tablespoon 3 times a day, 30 minutes before each meal until the entire amount is used up. Use this therapy once a year.

A recipe for "the elixir of youth", a type of garlic extract, was found in1971 by a UNESCO team in a Tibetan monastery and was dated about 4-5 centuries BC. The extract cleans accumulated fat out of the body, rinses out insoluble calcium, radically improves metabolism, cleanses blood vessels, prevents heart attacks, arteriosclerosis, and paralysis, removes the sensation of buzzing from the head, improves sight, and regenerates the entire body.

Remedy #29 (Garlic extract)
Take 12oz (350g) of peeled, freshly harvested garlic, crush it into a pulp, and mix with 7 fl oz (200mL) of vodka (40% proof and up). Close tightly in a jar and put in a dark, cool

place (do not refrigerate) for 10 days. Then strain the pulp, put the fluid in a jar and keep it in a dark place for another 4 days. Now it is ready.

Use the extract according to the following dosage:

Day	Breakfast	Lunch	Dinner
1	1 drop	2 drops	3 drops
2	4 drops	5 drops	6 drops
3	7 drops	8 drops	9 drops
4	10 drops	11 drops	12 drops
5	13 drops	14 drops	15 drops
6	16 drops	17 drops	18 drops
7	19 drops	20 drops	21 drops
8	22 drops	23 drops	24 drops
9	25 drops	25 drops	25 drops
10	25 drops	25 drops	25 drops
11	25 drops	25 drops	25 drops

After this, take 25 drops three times a day until all extract is used up. Each amount of the extract should be taken with 1.7 fl oz (50mL) of plain yogurt or kefir.

Many people dislike the intensive smell of garlic. To get rid of the smell, chew on a piece of parsley, an apple, a lemon peel, or an orange peel.

Caution - Use the garlic extract therapy only once a year.

The following remedy is also very effective in lowering cholesterol level.

Remedy #30

Warm up 1.8 oz (50g) of olive oil, put it in a cup, and squeeze juice out of a whole grapefruit into it. Drink the mixture, cover your liver area with a thermal pad, and lie down on your right side for 45-60 minutes. Don't eat anything for 2 hours. Repeat this routine for seven days in a row every 3 months. It is best to do it before going to bed, at least 3 hours after your last meal.

Avoid taking pills

A man who wasn't able to get out of bed because of terrible back pain once contacted me, looking for help. He told me he had read one of my books while on holidays and was amazed at how little he knew about his own body. Trying to alleviate pain, he decided to ask me for advice instead of taking painkillers. He had a doctor's appointment scheduled in a few days. I recommended an old, well tested method - sucking plant oil. Three days later, he was out of bed and all pain was gone.

Whenever there is an alternative method of solving a health problem, pharmaceutical drugs should be avoided. According to World Health Organization 30% of people over 50 have suffer from some kind of allergy to pharmaceuticals. Many elderly with a wide range of health problems have to take medications only to alleviate side effects of other medications. This usually causes damage to the stomach and liver. To avoid that, the following remedy can be tried against some health problems.

This remedy can be used in the treatment of vein inflammations, chronic anemia, paralysis, eczema, swelling, gastrointestinal disorders, heart and circulatory disorders, cancers, joint disorders, and many other health conditions, which may be less serious but still troublesome.

The method is simple, painless, and absolutely harmless. Many generations of Siberian healers used it with good effects.

Remedy #31

The therapy should be done on an empty stomach in the morning or before bedtime in the evening (3-4 hours after your last meal). Use not more than 1 tablespoon of sunflower oil or peanut oil, hold it in the front part of your mouth, and perform with your mouth, for 25-30 minutes, an action similar to sucking on a candy. The sucking action should not be very intense. The oil will thicken first and then it will become more liquid and white. Make sure you spit the oil out after the procedure. It should not be swallowed because it contains substances that can cause many diseases. You can use the method as long as needed. Eventually you will feel refreshed, energetic, and calm. You will also regain good sleep and memory. Acute diseases are cured quickly, within 2-3 weeks. Chronic conditions take several months to a year and we should be aware that the therapy might trigger certain mild symptoms (e.g. the feeling of weakness) during the first week. This phenomenon is associated with the weakening of the disease's focal points. It is normal and we need to go through the experience. Properly implemented therapy will bring such noticeable signs as more energy on awakening, better appetite, and the feeling of freshness. Based on the state of your health, you can make your own decision about the duration of the therapy. Healthy people and children can use the method for two weeks as a preventative measure. This will not only prevent diseases mentioned above but also remove toxic heavy metals that can be found even in a healthy body. I don't need to convince anybody that prevention is better than treatment. The method brings best results if used daily for 1-6 months.

Plant-based oils

People tend to have extreme opinions about the value of sun-flower oil: some don't have any use for it while others believe it to be a panacea against all health troubles. I'm strongly convinced that plant-based oils are a necessary part of our diet. They should equal about 50% of our entire fat intake (2-2oz/ 60-80g a day). They contain biologically active substances that help lower cholesterol level in our blood, preventing blood vessels from developing arteriosclerosis. This is important even for young people - many people under 20 years of age have higher than normal cholesterol level. They should limit animal fat intake and replace it with plant oils.

The advantage of plant oils over animal fats comes, among others, from the fact that they contain two unsaturated fatty acids - linoleic and linolenic, that our body can get only from food. They are essential for our body because they play a role in the synthesis of many hormones and hormone-like substances. Women going through menopause need at least 0.005-0.20oz (2-6g) of unsaturated fatty acids daily. Such amount is contained in 0.30-0.50oz (10-15g) of plant oil. However, to make sure we get adequate amounts of those acids, it's best for everybody to take 0.80-1oz (25-30g or 1-2 tablespoons) a day.

Many elderly people try to take large amounts of plant oils to stop the progression of arteriosclerosis. This can lead to irritation of the stomach and bile-secreting system. It's best to take oils in their raw form (e.g. in salads) because high temperature causes oxidation of fatty acids and the loss of their beneficial properties. The nutritional value of plant oils is so high that, combined with fish and eggs, they can replace meat and animal fats in our diet without making us deficient in any essential substances.

Sunflower oil - one of the most commonly used - is also one of the most valuable in terms of nutrition. Soy and peanut oil contain more unsaturated fatty acids, but they in turn are lower in vitamin and mineral content. Sunflower and olive oil are best in salads. Olive oil has neutral taste and practically no smell. It's very commonly used even though relatively poor in vitamins and other biologically active compounds. Corn oil has lower vitamin content than sunflower oil, but it's high in vitamin E and wonderfully reduces blood cholesterol level. Thanks to its unique makeup, corn oil has long been used in dealing with many health problems, most effectively in treating skin conditions.

Remedy #32

If your skin becomes flaky, you can take one tablespoon of corn oil once a day for a month (best with your breakfast or supper). In eczema cases in the form of dry flaky skin, you can take one teaspoon of corn oil with your breakfast and supper for two months. The downside of this therapy is its long duration, but the effect is permanent - eczema shouldn't bother you again and your skin will become smooth and re-juvenated.

Whenever I recommended oil therapy in my non-conventional practice, the effects were usually very good.

One of my patients was a twelve-year-old girl with half of her face swollen. Nobody knew the cause of swelling and creams that had been prescribed weren't bringing any results. I recommended taking two tablespoons of corn oil every day before going to bed. A month later the swelling disappeared as suddenly as it first showed up.

Another patient was a soldier whose hair started falling out as if it were dying, supposedly because of service-related stress.

He wasn't even able to comb his hair straight and the entire scalp was covered with dandruff. No shampoos proved effective, which didn't surprise me because the cause of any disorder has to be found and corrected in our own body. In this case, the cause was long-lasting improper nutrition and stress was the factor that triggered the unfortunate condition. I prescribed the following treatment:

Remedy #33

Take 1.8oz (50g) of corn oil mixed with 100mL of freshly squeezed grapefruit juice every other day before going to bed for two weeks. In addition, take a tablespoon of corn oil with your breakfast and supper.

My patient's hair became shiny again in less than a month. Dandruff disappeared completely. He remarked that he had never had such healthy and thick hair in his entire life.

Some practical advice:

1. Store plant oils tightly closed in a cool and dark place. Don't store for longer than six months.
2. Unrefined oils are better than refined ones.
3. Oil in glass bottles is better quality than the one stored in plastic containers.
4. It's normal to see a little sediment at the bottom of the container. These are biologically active substances found in oil.
5. Do not reuse oil in your frying pan. Don't fry your food very long. Prolong heat causes oil to form harmful compounds, which irritate the stomach and intestines, damage the liver, and lead to formation of cancer cells.

*We need to know our enemies to fight
them effectively.*

Reverse Cancer

I've had many opportunities to witness the situation when even strong-spirited people suddenly paled having heard the terrible diagnosis - cancer. Everyone was accepting this news like the death sentence without any possibility for appeal. Despite seeming hopelessness of their situation, even seriously ill people with incurable diseases try to hold on to life to the very last moments. This is in our human nature - we fully appreciate health only after we lose it. Today's medicine isn't able to give full answers about the causes of cancer. What force directs some cells to mutate, rapidly reproduce, and grow into healthy tissue causing a lot of pain and suffering? Doctors and researchers have created a lot of theories explaining the mechanism of tumor formation and identified many factors stimulating the development of cancer cells. However, they haven't managed to find the original cause. I think that the research failed for the following reasons:

First, cancer research treats the human body as a set of organs instead of looking at it as a biological system. All efforts concentrate on the ill organ where a tumor is discovered. The usual treatment - radiation and chemotherapy - is theoretically intended to mobilize the body's defense mechanisms. Unfortunately, the body is weakened by the disease and poisoned from within. As such, it doesn't have any reserves to come up with effective defense. The treatment itself creates another disadvantage by making bodily fluids more alkaline, which promotes the growth of unhealthy bacteria posing more challenge to our immune system.

Second, medicine keeps looking for a universal drug or a combination of drugs to effectively reverse the growth of tumors (fighting the symptoms not the cause), while cancer is a disease involving the whole body, from the brain to the large intestine.

The "seeds" of cancer are ingrained in us from our childhood. They start "sprouting" as transitional stages of the underlying disease. Runny nose, colds, rheumatism, arthritis, and other conditions affecting our eyes, ears, throat, kidneys, liver, heart, bones, or the nervous system, are all segments of one cancerous chain. As long as we don't create proper circumstances allowing our body to utilize it's natural defense mechanisms involving immunity, self-regulation, and self-regeneration, thousands of research centers and millions of doctors with all the drugs and other methods will be unsuccessful in their efforts to cure cancer. Even patients who have a successful surgery and get good prognosis still have a constant unconscious fear of recurrence.

I've been in contact with a lot of cancer patients for many years. There are thousands of them in hospitals all over the world. Many stay alive despite the odds. One of them was a 39-year-old woman who came to see me in the Health Center in Moscow. She had been diagnosed with pancreatic cancer. Two surgeries in the course of six months left her very weak and she was given 2-3 months to live. She had constant 100-102F (38-39C) fever and her vitality was visibly diminishing.

I said to her: "There are three of us - you, me, and your disease. Who do you want to align with? Two can always defeat one." She didn't say anything but the expression in her eyes proved she was ready to fight to the end.

The first step in the treatment was large intestine cleaning with the use of enema. This method was first introduced in 1946 by Dr. Max Gerson, an American physician. It was used with good results for many years in the cancer clinic run by Dr. Gerson's daughter. Since many modern doctors treat enema as something obsolete, its use in cancer therapy was eventually discontinued and forgotten.

The essence of this method is performing 6-8 enemas a day. The irrigation solution is 1.5qt (1.5L) of boiled water up to 100F (38C) warm mixed with 3-4 teaspoons of lemon juice and a cup of beet juice. The number of enemas in the first stage depends on the condition of the patient - more enemas are used for cases that are more serious. In the next stage, an enema is used once a day or once every other day until the patient starts producing spontaneous stools.

The therapeutic effect of this procedure can be explained this way: Intestinal cleansing helps eliminate toxins that are produced by cancer cells in their life processes. If these toxins are not removed, they get into the blood stream and are carried all over the body, blocking the body's self-regulatory mechanisms and leading to death.

In 1950-ies, Dr. Gerson pointed out to his students that the functioning of our large intestine is closely related with the function of the brain and central nervous system. According to him, cancer is our body's vengeance for improperly eaten meals. In 99% of the cases we invite cancer by poisoning ourselves, only 1% is caused by spontaneous changes in our body. This means that we are 1% victims and 99% authors of cancer.

If a cancerous tumor attacks the digestive tract, the choice of diet is an important task. Meat, fish, dairy products, broth and other soups are not recommended. We are left with grains, fruits, and vegetables. Combining fruits and vegetables, either raw or cooked, is improper because they require different digestive times - 2 hours for fruits and 4 hours for vegetables. We can, however, drink any combinations of freshly squeezed fruit and vegetable juices because they are absorbed in practically the same time. They provide large amounts of essential vitamins, minerals, and hormones without the necessity to spend our body's energy in digestive processes. My patient, while using enemas, was able to eat only rice, buckwheat, and baked potatoes. She also drank about 2qt (2L) of juices every day.

Beet and carrot juices play a special role in cancer therapy (see "Can We Live 150 Years?" pages 85-86). Scientific studies conducted over many years proved that these juices slow down the growth of tumors, flush out old cancer cells, and enhance the functioning of respiratory enzymes (beet juice can increase the enzyme functioning by 400-1000%). The role of pigments contained in beets and carrots is not exactly known, however they've been proven by research to slow down the development of cancer cells.

The best combination for cancer patients is a 4:1 blend of carrot juice and beet juice. Every day, 1-2qt (1-2L) of juice blend should be used in equal amounts, with 4-hour intervals during the day, plus one portion at 1 a.m. Some people cannot tolerate beet juice and react with nausea, weakness, slow heart rate, and low blood pressure. In such cases, we have to limit the amount to two tablespoons a day and gradually increase it day after day. We can also substitute beet juice with apple juice, adding two tablespoons of red wine per one liter of blend.

Experts have different opinions about whether beet juice should be consumed freshly squeezed or after 1-1.5 hours. Freshly squeezed beet juice contains 2.5 times more active oxygen and active iron, which is essential for hemoglobin. This is why it's better for cancer patients to drink freshly squeezed beet juice. I would say it's also necessary for elderly people whose cellular breathing is impaired. Regular use of beet juice guarantees a rejuvenated body, healthy white teeth, and 80% protection against cancer.

Cancer attacks not only our body but also the mind. This is why I asked my patient to spend considerable time on exercises stabilizing her psychological condition. Since she wasn't able to relax and release her strong nervous tension, I had to teach her self-hypnosis. We also went together through ten hypnotic regressions, taking her back to her childhood experiences (For many people, cancer is a result of trauma in early childhood.) We dealt, step by step, with psychological "roots" that kept her disease alive. She hadn't had a happy childhood: her father had abused alcohol and beaten her and her mother. She hadn't had toys or been allowed to bring friends home. Overall, it wasn't a pretty picture. Her adult life wasn't easy either. It seemed that she could achieve anything only with great difficulty. She blamed it all on her parents, especially the father who had done her a lot of injustice in her childhood.

I tried to convince her during those hypnotic sessions that holding a grudge "consumes" our body and finally leads to cancer. If anger and hatred dominate our feelings, we burn out from inside. Such emotions don't usually go together with good health.

The next stage in her therapy was teaching her self-healing method in order to fully release her body's potential defense mechanisms that remain inactive in most people all their life.

The pharmacy inside our own body (self-healing method)

Nature provided each one of us with an excellent individual "pharmacy" containing medicine against all diseases we can ever get. Our only task is learning how to make use of it.

The self-healing process has two stages. The first stage is relaxing all the muscles in our body. In the second stage, we launch a healing program in our subconscious mind (just like a computer program) designed to trigger our body's self-regulatory processes. Self-healing is effective because it uses our body's natural defense mechanisms.

Stage 1 - relaxing

Spread a soft blanket on the floor and lie down on your back. Your arms should be stretched alongside your body with the palms facing outside and the fingers slightly bowed, your feet tilted outside, your head turned to one side, mouth open, tongue against the upper teeth, and your eyes closed for better concentration. Try to be calm, not to think about anything, and, most important of all, breathe calmly and evenly. It usually takes two to five minutes to achieve full relaxation state.

Stage 2 - self-healing

The cells in our body have a basic mental capability similar to that of a little child. We should remember that fact when we address an ill organ. In your imagination try to visualize the malfunctioning organ, open communication with it, and concentrate on giving it an order. The order must be expressed clearly and decisively, as if you were trying to correct the behavior of your beloved child.

Each one of our organs has its own "personality," for example our stomach and our liver are stubborn and not very reasonable. They need to be addressed in the form of a harsh command. Our heart is much wiser and it listens to requests expressed gently and cordially.

Having completed the first stage you can, for example, imagine looking inside your heart and try to see a small bright flame in it - the source of love and saving energy. Imagine that the flame grows, fills your whole heart, and then spreads throughout the entire body from the top of your head to the tips of your fingers and toes. Try to feel how it cleanses your body, removes inflammations, and brings health and vigor. Quietly say to yourself: "Every breath brings me closer to full cleansing. The light in my body is the healing energy."

If you know a specific spot with a lump or inflammation, put your right hand on it and imagine that the healing light is emitted from the center of your palm and it melts the lump just like sunrays melt snow or ice in the spring.

This was just an example. Everybody has enough imagination to develop his or her own healing scenario. The most important thing to remember is to relax your muscles and to enter the healing program into your subconscious mind. You can pick any time for self-healing sessions but it's done better when there is nobody around to interrupt you. If you enjoy quiet music, turn on your favorite piece for a better relaxation effect.

Both people with cancer and their caretakers have to understand that the patients' optimism, love for life and faith in the possibility of healing play the decisive role in victory over the disease. In much too many cases, ill people become passive observers expecting miraculous help from doctors. Such patients lie passively in bed, refuse to take action, and worry to death despite being told hundreds of times about the possibilities of modern medicine and the importance of not giving up. As long as patients' own attitude doesn't change, such "psychotherapy" coming from other sources has no effect.

Surgical removal of tumors is an invasive procedure involving our body's complex structures. In many cases, it can be compared to an attempt on repairing an electronic device with the use of a hammer and a crowbar. It's often the last resort, when we run out of other options. If the surgeons find out that nothing can be done, the patient is stitched up and sent home to die. Sometimes the patient doesn't even know the terrible truth, only the immediate family. Wouldn't it be better to be honest instead of putting on a spectacle? This would allow the ill person to consider something else that could turn out to be the last chance. It may seem cruel, but truth cannot be cruel. It doesn't kill. Truth can heal if the affected person finds enough courage and strength to face and understand it.

People ignored the principles of moderate eating and physical exercise. They poison their lungs and blood with cigarette smoke, drinking too much coffee, and eating excessive amounts of sweets. All this puts a lot of strain on our body's defenses. Our body begs for some cooperation by sending us different signals, but we ignore them or silence them with various pills. There is time when the only option is listening to our tired body's signals and helping it recover. It's a chance to prolong our life and it's up to us to use it.

Going back to my female patient, she had to work on herself quite a bit before she got cured. On top of all methods I just described, she went through four liver-cleansing routines, took various herbal baths, used aerobic and aquatic therapies, exercised a lot (including some specific exercises for cancer patients), followed a special diet, and drank herbal teas (raspberry, black currant, nettle). After six months of intensive work on her health, she went to see the doctor who had written her

off. He could only say, "You are alive after all. I thought..."
I'd like everybody to stick to the following principles, no matter how grave your health condition becomes:

1. Believe you have enough strength to fight the disease.
2. Never abandon hope for recovery.
3. Love your body and mind.

Everybody should understand that cancer is the final link in a long chain of diseases. It's not an illness of one single organ but of all systems in our body, one of which gives in first. Cancer is, first of all, a result of unhealthy lifestyle, inability to handle stress, ignorance of our physiology, and disregard for the laws of nature.
Efforts concentrated on fighting specific tumors have little chance of success. Cancer kills well-known politicians, movie stars, and other celebrities, even though they have enough money to afford the most expensive treatments. It's an unavoidable result of the lifestyle most people live. The seeds of cancer exist in everybody from the time we are born (it's in the genetic memory of infants). It takes time for the disease to develop and manifest itself. Many people don't live long enough - they die earlier of other diseases. It's most often diagnosed in rich, well-developed economically countries. However, even early detection doesn't guarantee cure if we don't take radical steps in changing the lifestyle. Statistics in well-developed countries doesn't give much reason for hope despite modern medical equipment, availability of pharmaceuticals, and high level of medical training - one out of four Americans die of cancer. People living in underdeveloped countries simply don't live long enough to develop cancer. They die of earlier diseases, such as heart attack, stroke, and the like.

What do people get ill with and quickly die of

Trying to research the formation process of many diseases doesn't require as much time as we might think. Even though every person's body is as unique as our fingerprints, the general outline of disease process is roughly the same. In simple terms, every health problem, from a simple rush or allergy to cancer on one of our organs, is a disorder of the whole body. Whatever name we give it, its cause is the accumulation of toxins. The toxins come from two sources:

1. From outside with food, air, water, medications, etc.
2. Produced in our body as a result of its own life processes and life processes of bacteria living in it.

Undigested food forms deposits in the large intestine and becomes breeding ground for toxin-producing bacteria. Toxins are absorbed by intestinal walls and blood carries them to all our organs, where they cause diseases. To make the point, I'll use a drastic example of experiments done by the Nazis during the Second World War. They took the contents of the large intestine from prisoners suffering from chronic constipation, made serum from it, and injected healthy prisoners with it. Depending on the amount of serum, the injections resulted in psychological disorders, burst blood vessels, and strokes.

Professor Zepp of Moscow University wrote at the beginning of the twentieth century an interesting book that was never published, like many other works written by Russian doctors. He found out in his experiments that stroke is caused by ear inflammation, which in turn is a result of throat inflammation. The throat gets ill because the kidneys don't function properly. Kidneys malfunction because people use bedding that is to warm and wear warm air tight clothing. Kidney disease distorts skin breathing and other skin function. Poor functioning of skin and kidneys leads to liver disease, and these are followed by irregularities in circulatory and digestive systems. Resulting constipation causes autotoxication (self-poisoning) in the body, accompanied by headaches. Blood vessels in the brain expand and are ready to burst. When a blood vessel bursts (micro-stroke), the damage done in the brain can affect all bodily systems and can result in psychosis, schizophrenia, dementia, hearing impairment, vision disorders, large intestine disorders, gallbladder and kidney stones, rheumatism, etc.

At about the same time in another part of the world, Japanese professor Nishi noticed that 99% of people that die of various diseases have micro-strokes in those sections of the brain that direct the movement of limbs. This led him to an explanation for the phenomenon of cold hands and feet. People with constantly cold hands and feet suffer from disorders in the functioning of the heart, blood vessels, and kidneys. Their lungs and liver are also inefficient, and all this is caused by frequent constipation. When food isn't fully digested and absorbed, undigested pieces decompose in the large intestine. One of the products is carbon monoxide. It binds with hemoglobin to produce a toxic compound, which accumulates and causes damage to our body, especially the circulatory system. Nishi concluded that brain and large intestine are the most important organs in the body.

Abbot, an American doctor, published a study before the Second World War in which he tied the origin of some diseases to changes in the spine. (See "An ill spine means an ill body" at page 16 of "Can We Live 150 Years?")

Various body movements can often cause minute dislocations of vertebrae; the muscles around a dislocated vertebra stiffen up and prevent it from moving back to its proper position. This results in progressive nerve and muscle inflammation, causing pain and limiting our range of motion.

A dislocated vertebra creates pressure on nerves and blood vessels that are connected with specific muscles and organs. If a nerve remains under pressure for a long time, the organ depending on that nerve develops pathologies that are hard to cure.

The following health problems are associated with dislocations in corresponding spinal sections:

Cervical - Allergies, loss of hearing, sight problems, eczema, throat problems, thyroid gland disorders;

Thoracic - Asthma, pain in the lower arms, back pains, gall bladder disorders, liver problems, stomach and duodenum ulcers, kidney diseases, skin disorders (acne, rashes, eczema, boils);

Lumbar - Hemorrhoids, bladder disorders, irregular menstrual cycle, menstrual pains, impotence, knee pain, lumbago, lumbar pain, poor blood circulation in the legs, ankle swelling, cold feet, weak legs, muscular cramps in the legs.

All health disorders reflect unhealthy lifestyle - wrong diet, improper breathing, poor sleep, lack of exercise, and negative thinking - we lead from our childhood to old age. The long chain of health problems can originate from minute changes in the spine caused by incorrect sleeping position and lack of exercise. These changes can lead to impairment in skin function and deficiency of oxygen in the body. The process intensifies if we dress too warmly and neglect aerobic and aquatic exercises.

Inefficient skin breathing negatively influences the function of liver and kidneys (stones, low filtering abilities) and also negatively changes the composition of blood.

Poor blood quality can cause vein disorders, muscle cramps in the legs, tooth decay, poor condition of hair and nails, inefficiency of the heart, problems with eyes, ears, and finally with the brain.

Inefficiency in liver and kidney function leads to gastrointestinal disorders (indigestion, heartburn) and to stomach and duodenum diseases. On top of that, it leads to chronic constipation and resulting autotoxication, accompanied by nerve and psychological disorders, headaches, weakness, insomnia, and finally broken blood vessels in the brain. Even if it doesn't result in death, it paralyzes our limbs by damaging the brain area responsible for directing our movements.

Paralyzed and cold limbs negatively affect the condition of our heart, blood vessels, and kidneys. We face the possibility of heart disease, cancer, or Alzheimer's disease. It becomes a closed circle.

The order of disease development can of course be different for everybody. The specific "scenario" is an individual thing. Sometimes diseases develop simultaneously. You can use your own example or that of a relative or friend to analyze the connection between lifestyle and the state of health.

We breed cancer ourselves

One of my patients was a twelve-year-old boy who had been suffering from asthmatic fits for the last two years. His face was swollen and skin complexion yellowish-pale. As a result of hormonal therapy, he was considerably overweight and was not able to participate in physical activities at school. I noticed spinal misalignment. He could only dream about such things as playing ball, cycling, or swimming.

There he was in front of me, an unhappy twelve-year-old who couldn't enjoy his childhood and was almost handicapped. And his future seemed to look even bleaker than that because bronchial asthma is a chronic and hard-to-cure disease. Questioned about his favorite foods, his mother mentioned meat, soups, dairy products, pastry, and sweets.

I could never understand parents who in their blind affection treat children with candies, ice cream, sweet beverages, and other products that are full of sugar. They don't realize that all these products turn into poisons and remain in their children's bodies for the rest of their lives. When I hear discussions about hereditary diseases, I often want to say that diseases are not inherited. We inherit an unhealthy lifestyle.

I asked another question, about his morning exercises and other hardiness-building activities. It turned out he didn't have any such habits. Many children today are affected by obesity, vision disorders, and infections because they spend most of their free time watching TV or playing computer games instead of playing outdoors.

I further questioned the boy's mother:

"How does he like to sleep?"
"Soft mattress, high pillow, thick warm quilt..."
"Does he often get sore throat or flu?"
"Yes."
"Does he have regular stools?" - She shrugged her shoulders.
"I don't really know."
I questioned the boy about bowel movements, which caused him to blush.

"I do it with difficulty and it's in the form of hard round chunks."
"How often do you get headaches?"
"At least once a week."
"What do you do then?"
"Nothing. I lie in bed or Mom gives me a pill..."
He was a child, somebody just starting his life, and from

what I heard about his lifestyle, he was already a potential candidate for a cancer patient. According to statistics, in the western world one child out of four has respiratory disorders, one out of five - gastrointestinal disorders, one out of five - vision and hearing disorders, and one out of three - neurological disorders. Many children suffer from constipation and headaches. It's almost impossible to find a completely healthy child. What's going to happen when they become adults?

Nature takes care of those who live in harmony with her laws. When babies are born, they breathe air in and soon get a bath - their first contact with water. Soon after, they are exposed to sunlight and come in contact with the ground. Dying people say farewell to sunlight, stop breathing and get buried in the ground. What happens between birth and death is closely related to sunlight, air, water, and earth. Sun gives us energy, air provides oxygen, water fills our cells, and the land feeds us. These laws of nature are constant and universal.

Humans don't want to live according to the laws of nature and are getting illness and suffering in return. We started creating artificial environments and avoiding sunlight. We poisoned our air and water and replaced natural food with attractively wrapped processed products. We want all our food to be tasty, sweet, cooked, and warm. Nutritional value of such processed food is usually depleted. Our natural hardiness got watered down. Polluted blood carries disease-causing poisons, the heart gets weakened and the brain damaged. No pills are going to help when our body resembles a dirty stagnant swamp. We have a choice between disease bringing a premature death or changing our lifestyle and enjoying vibrant health. An old adage teaches, "doctors treat and nature heals." Our body can deal with any disease if we create conditions allowing it to utilize its natural defenses.

Cancer-preventing Nishi system

In my practice with cancer patients, an essential element of treatment was always Nishi therapeutic system. It's not as impressive as complex radiation equipment and other sophisticated hardware supporting surgical teams in modern operating rooms, but it brings good results nevertheless. I'm going to present a few examples of successful use of Nishi system (records of professor Watanabe), to let you see for yourself.

- K. Majra, 76 years, was diagnosed with lung cancer in August 1958. He didn't consent to a surgery. Another test in a Tokyo hospital confirmed the diagnosis. He was treated in hospital for two months, which caused general weakening, gradual loss of appetite, and severe difficulties with breathing. An X-ray picture done in the second month of his hospital stay showed the same dark spot on the lungs and an enlarged one in the heart area. This last one was a side effect of pharmaceuticals that interfered with blood and lymph circulation. Breathing became almost impossible. There seemed to be no options, even a surgery would give no chances. He was checked out of hospital in December. Some relative suggested trying Nishi system. He used the following routines every day:

  1. Aerobic therapy
  2. Alternating hot and cold showers
  3. Drinking beverage prepared from dactyl palm leaves, very rich in vitamin C (2qt /2L a day)
  4. Performing a set of exercises designed by Dr. Nishi

After a month, his appetite increased, his physical strength returned, breathing became easier, and his mood improved. The dark spot on his lungs, as big as a chicken egg, started shrinking. A year later (November 1959) the patient was completely healthy. He decided to use cancer-preventing Nishi system till the end of his life.

- T. Jumiki, 69 years old, after a thorough examination in hospital was found to have stomach cancer. A surgery was recommended, and he refused consent. He decided to go through Nishi system therapy.

A month of therapy decreased nausea and took care of the feeling of discomfort in the stomach. A year later in a letter, he reported that he felt well. He was thankful for the therapy that cured his stomach cancer without surgery.

- Iszizuko, 61 years old, in the summer 1958 started experiencing pain in his abdomen while having his meals. His stools were dark because of blood mixed with the feces. Doctors in an Osaka hospital diagnosed colon cancer. He refused a surgery and checked into another hospital where he learned Nishi system therapy, which eventually led him to full recovery.

- Masapugu, 68 years old, lost his ability to speak and was diagnosed with throat cancer by doctors in Osaka. Isotope radiation therapy didn't bring any improvement. He checked into a hospital for Nishi system therapy in November 1958. He had unhealthy habits - smoking up to forty cigarettes a day and eating a lot of sweets. These habits caused even more irritation in the affected area of his throat. Two months of therapy brought significant improvement and his voice became normal. He was able to check out of the hospital and continue the therapy on his own. In 1962, he sent a letter thanking the hospital for help in his full return to health.

- Gojono Sato, 49 years old, suffered heavy bleeding from uterus for five years due to uterus cancer. She checked into a hospital for eight months to undergo Nishi system therapy. The first results were noticed at the end of the second month: her physical condition improved and heavy bleeding carried out chunks of dead tissue. She checked out of the hospital at that time and continued the therapy at home with some help in the form of telephone consultations. Bleedings with chunks of dead tissue happened on three more occasions. Examinations after completed therapy confirmed her return to good health. The doctor who first recommended surgery was amazed at her recovery and said: "You are very lucky. The diagnosis was probably wrong."

These were cases from 40 years ago. Nishi system therapy is however successfully used in Japan even today for cancer treatment. Starting in 1990, many alternative medicine clinics in Russia started using it in their practice.

I have been using it, along with my co-workers, since 1986, with some modifications (to account for different climate, food products, etc.) I didn't keep statistics because the patients had medical records anyway, but I kept letters from my patients reporting results of their therapy done at home. I'll summarize some cases here:

Natalia D., 44 years old, was diagnosed in 1986 with uterus cancer, which had also spread to her breast. Her doctor first pressed for a quick surgery. She was in bad shape, with grayish skin complexion, bent posture, and an unpleasant odor from her mouth. Faced with her hesitation, the doctor agreed to delay the surgery for eight weeks. He understood the 44-year-old woman's shock at the prospect of loosing her reproductive organs and breasts. Natalia kept working but her husband took over her house chores (it's important to have support and understanding of loved ones in times of health crisis). She went through therapy involving aerobics twice a day; drinking tea brewed from blackcurrant leaves, raspberry, and wild rose; taking alternating hot and cold showers; and performing a set of exercises from Nishi system. She also cleansed her large intestine using enemas and limited her diet to raw fruits, nuts, bran, rice, hot cereals with cooked vegetables, carrot juice, and beet juice.

Three weeks later, her skin was covered with red spots and her vagina excreted "terrible filth." It was a sign that her body started cleaning itself. Then she went through a seven-day fast. She only drank water, adding a teaspoon of apple cider vinegar and a teaspoon of honey to each glass in order to maintain adequate supply of minerals and vitamins. After a fast, the body needs an adjustment period of equal length before regular diet can be re-introduced. For the next seven days, she only drank freshly squeezed juices from five kinds of fruits and vegetables of different colors, and ate only fruits and vegetables.

In her later diet, she paid attention to correct combination of food products. She fearfully went back to see her doctor when the eight-week period was up. After the examination, not able to hide his disbelief, the doctor said, "I can't believe my eyes, haw did you do it?" After hearing the story of her quick and effective therapy, he exclaimed: "I have to tell everybody about it."

I got her letter a year after the end of the therapy. She felt healthy, continued working, and enjoyed her life.

In matters dealing with health, some of us are lazy (please take no offence) and some diligent. The lazy ones expect others to help them. They believe that taking care of their health is the responsibility of physicians. The diligent ones want to help themselves by discovering the real causes of their diseases but they do not always know how to do it. My books are intended mainly for the diligent people. The lazy ones should reflect on the old Eastern wisdom: "Nobody does anything for you without satisfying their own needs before yours." You ought not to thoughtlessly leave your most valuable things - your life and health - in somebody else's care. We spend our time in vain while we wait for a miraculous healing coming from somebody else - nobody can take better care of our health than ourselves. It takes strong will, persistency, diligence, knowledge, and experience to find our own way to good health. As we know, those who seek will always find.

Modern medicine uses three basic methods in treating cancer: chemotherapy, radiation, and surgery. As I said before, these methods are limited to treating symptoms. The right approach is to identify and target causes. According to our present knowledge, the main cause of tumors is inability of our body's defenses to effectively deal with cancer cells. This is where prevention and treatment should be focused.

The complex system I'm going to present here has never undergone scientific scrutiny. It can only be judged based on the testimony of people who suffered from cancer, managed to overcome it, and are now completely healthy. It was never published, but my students and co-workers may have used some elements. Important notice: **The system can be used independently of other treatments and medications taken. Its strength is in mobilizing body's own defenses.** The "downside" is the fact that it requires from patients ongoing focus on caring for their health. The system takes more time to show results in serious cases, lighter ones can be dealt with relatively quickly. Those who go through the therapy learn a way to maintain good health for the rest of their lives.

The system was designed based on:

1. The works of Ivan Pavlov, a Russian physiologist, proposing the thesis that human body is a self-regulating, self-curing, self-sustaining, regenerating, and improving system
2. The works of Ugolev, a Russian expert in the area of digestion
3. The works of Dr. Norman Walker and Dr. Max Gerson in the area of cancer treatment
4. Body cleansing methods used by Tibetan healers
5. Hydrotherapy and other immunity-building methods proposed by S. Kneipp and Porfir Ivanov
6. Physical exercises designed by Dr. Katsuzo Nishi for cancer therapy
7. My own observations from unconventional medicine practice in Moscow Health Institute

Hippocrates said:

> *If diseases are part of natural order, nature has cures for them. We only have to find those cures.*

How can we do it? We have to live in harmony with the laws of nature. Here are some steps:

1. Learn breathing exercises ("Can We Live 150 Years?" page 74)
2. Change your nutritional habits ("Can We Live 150 Years?" page 103)
3. Drink freshly squeezed fruit and vegetable juices
4. Use aquatic immunity-building therapies (baths, sauna,

alternating hot and cold showers, ("Can We Live 150 Years?" page 94)
5. Increase your physical activities (p. 61-63, 65-67, 81-82).
6. Use body-cleansing routines ("Can We Live 150 Years?" page 177)
7. Perform Nishi cancer-preventing exercise set.
8. Learn to control your psychology (emotions, thoughts, and desires, (p. 98)

A wider description of all these points can be found throughout all my books. Here are a few pieces of advice concerning nutritional habits:

1. Gradually eliminate from your diet all refined and heavily processed food products (sausages, deli, margarine, canned food, spirit vinegar, white flour, instant soups, sauces, etc.)
2. Limit as much as possible your intake of sugar and products containing sugar or its dietary substitutes (use honey instead).
3. Limit as much as possible your intake of stimulants (coffee, black tea, hard liquor).
4. Eat as little as possible animal fats (butter, cheese, fatty meat).
5. Limit to a minimum your consumption of yeast containing baked goods.

Your diet can include cereals, cooked rice (best unrefined), fruits and vegetables (at least five kinds, both cooked and raw), fish, poultry, wheat sprouts, cheese (1-2 slices a day, and eggs (soft - 3 times a week).

When planning your menu, use the following rules: **Eat food produced by the land, best grown in your geogra-**

phical region, raw or cooked, honey, eggs, and sour milk.
Take into account the principles of correctly combining food
products (Table 2, p. 52). Here is some more advice concerning your meals:

> ➢ The proper order is juice, salad, and the main course. Eat
> carbohydrates (cereals, potatoes, fruits, vegetables, and
> other plant-based products) before noon and proteins (fish,
> cheese, other animal products) in the afternoon.
> ➢ It's best to eat two meals a day. If you feel hungry in the
> meantime, eat fruits and vegetables or drink tea brewed
> from raspberry, blackberry, birch, or blackcurrant leaves.
> ➢ Chew each bite thoroughly (25-30 times for healthy
> people, 50-70 times for ill people).
> ➢ Drink freshly squeezed fruit and vegetable juices and eat
> salads before your meals.

One of the most important discoveries of the twentieth century in the area of nutrition was a new digestion theory. According to this theory, besides the stomach and the small intestine,
blood vessels also take part in the digestion process. This is
why incorrect nutrition violating basic principles is sure to cause
health problems.

The old idea that the small intestine produces only one stream of nutrients was proven wrong by Ugolev who showed that
there are at least five of them. One of the streams carries over
thirty hormones and other hormone-like substances, which are
produced by the intestine and its bacterial flora and play cru-
cial role not only in the digestive process but also other physiological functions in the entire body. The combined cellular
mass of the intestine and its flora is bigger than that of all endocrine glands and they produce identical kinds of hormones as
those produced by the endocrine system. On top of that, the

small intestine's microflora can produced essential hormones, vitamins, and amino-acids. This is why every disturbance in microflora development (e.g. due to the use of antibiotics) or creating circumstances for pathologies in its growth (e.g. resulting from overuse of refined and cooked food products) destroys the body's hormonal system.

By the way, the theory easily explains some of the common health problems, such as for example thyroid gland disorders. They are results of digestive irregularities. The main causes of thyroid problems are eating too fast, incorrectly combining food products, and drinking at meals. Try to change those habits and thyroid disorders will disappear.

It's obvious that pathologies most people suffer from come from disturbed microflora. The pathologies start in infancy if the baby is fed cow milk and its products instead of mother's breast milk. This replaces normal and healthy milk fermentation with putrefaction processes that poison the child's body and later result in allergies, runny nose, staphylococci infections, sinus problems, and hundreds of other health disorders. This is why we should drink freshly squeezed juices before every meal in order to strengthen our hormonal system and provide enough vitamins, minerals, macro-, and micro-elements. The juice should be followed by a salad from at least five different kinds of vegetables (e.g. potatoes, cabbage, beets, carrot, and onion). Such salad contains all necessary fibers and other bulky materials - important components of our food, necessary for normal functioning of our digestive system and the whole body. Deficiency of fiber in food leads to irregularities in cholesterol exchange and hormonal exchange; it also promotes formation of stones. Bacterial flora feeds on fiber and transforms it in vitamins and essential amino acids. They make our large intestine work and move food along. This is especially important because of sitting lifestyle many of us lead.

Fiber accelerates the removal of toxins from the body and helps in retaining needed ions of potassium, calcium, sodium, and magnesium. Fruits and vegetables are rich in fibers. This is why it's good to eat a lot of salads all year round. They are especially important for the elderly - there is no better way to prevent diabetes and obesity. Those who already lost their teeth (because of eating too much cooked and sweet food) can grate their fruits and vegetables on plastic grates or drink freshly squeezed juices containing pulp, so that they can get as much fiber as possible. You can significantly improve your health if you get into the habit of starting your meals that way. People who eat mainly sandwiches, soups, and meat have their appetite-regulating mechanism out of order. They constantly feel hungry. Overeating leads them to obesity and poisoning with undigested chunks of food.

Cancer-preventing Nishi system includes:

1. Sleeping on a firm mattress and a firm pillow;
2. Performing "fish" exercise: lie on your back, put your hands on the area of the fourth and the fifth cervical vertebra, bend your elbows, and keep your whole body as tight to the floor as possible. Join your legs and pull the toes towards your head. Push your head, shoulders, calves, and pelvis towards the floor. Now start quick movements, swinging your body left and right, like a fast swimming fish. Perform this exercise in the morning and in the evening, one minute each time. Despite its simplicity, the exercise produces amazing results in removing spinal misalignments. It moves vertebra back to their proper positions, removing pressure from affected blood vessels and nerve endings (pinched nerve endings are the cause of many diseases).

3. Cockroach exercise: Lie on your back, put a firm semi-cylindrical pillow under your neck, stretch your arms and legs up (high enough for your feet to be parallel to the floor). Shake your feet and arms, like a cockroach turned on its back. Exercise for 1-2 minutes every morning and evening. What's the secret of this exercise? Everybody knows about health benefits of running. "Cockroach" exercise gives the same effect without any strain on joints and heart, which is very important for people who are weak, have reduced mobility, or are bedridden. The exercise increases blood circulation in the body, especially in your limbs.

4. Joining palms and feet: This exercise has four steps. It helps bring energy balance in the body back to normal. A healthy person has the same electrical charge in the left and the right side of the body. Upsetting this balance can lead to disease (That's how diagnosis is made based on an aura). Step 1: Lie on your back, join and part your palms ten times, pushing hard the tips of your fingers against one another. Step 2: Put your palms together. With your arms parallel to the torso, then move your hands up and down your body, as if you were trying to cut it in half (10 times). Step 3: Put your feet next to each other, raise them, and move them back and forth 10 times, "cutting" with your hands at the same time as in step 2. Step 4: Lie down with eyes closed, your palms joined, and your feet next to each other for 3-5 minutes.

5. Exercises to regenerate your cervical vertebrae and improve breathing

   ➤ Sitting in a chair, raise and lower your arms 10 times.
   ➤ Tilt your head left and right 10 times, trying to reach the tops of your shoulders with your ears.

> ➢ Tilt your head back and forth 10 times.
> ➢ Turn your head left and right 10 times.
> ➢ Stretch your arms in front of you with the palms facing each other, then turn your head left and right 10 times.
> ➢ Stretch your arms above your head with the palms facing each other, then turn your head left and right 5 times.
> ➢ Put your fingers on top of your shoulders and push your elbows back as far as possible (Imagine that you are trying to squeeze an apple between your shoulder blades). At the same time, push your chin forward (like a swan stretching its neck). This exercise relaxes vertebrae and muscles in your neck, which in turn improves blood circulation in your brain and normalizes the functioning of your nervous and digestive system. Perform the exercise in the morning and in the evening, 3 minutes each time.
> ➢ Sitting on the edge of a chair, rest your hands on your knees, close your eyes, and rock your body left and right. At the same time, expand your abdomen and pull it back in, following the same rhythm.

I consider this exercise set the best of all I know for a few reasons. First, no other set rejuvenates all bodily systems to the same degree. Second, The Japanese are known for their ability to gather knowledge, including medical knowledge, from all parts of the world, and pick out the best things out of it. Third, Japanese statistical data prove high effectiveness of this set as part of anti-cancer therapy. Fourth, I rely on my personal experience with this exercise set, having used it to correct some serious spine problems and to regain good physical and psychological condition.

Beside all the steps mentioned above, there are some additional measures that can complement the therapy.

1. Suck vegetable oil (3-4 times a day).
2. Drink tea brewed from raspberry or currant leaves (about 1qt/1L a day).
3. Eat a ground up eggshell every day.
4. Eat a lot of foods rich in phyto-estrogens (soy beans, beans, cabbage, broccoli).
5. Add garlic, onions, radish, and mustard seeds to your meals. They contain natural antibiotics.
6. Eat a lot of sauerkraut and pickled cucumbers (good sources of vitamin C).
7. Include in your diet products that are rich in iron and copper (apples, strawberries, raspberries, beets, blackcurrant, and carrots).
8. Eat products containing selenium, zinc, phosphorus, magnesium, vitamin E and B (wheat sprouts, oats, barley cereal, millet, and bran).
9. Use iodine - a very useful substance for prevention and treatment (see remedy #34).

Remedy #34 (Increases immunity and promotes higher leukocyte count in the blood, activates leukocytes, lowers cholesterol level, cleanses blood vessels.)

Mix 1 teaspoon of iodine (for external use) with 50mL of warm boiled water, add a tablespoon of potato flour (starch), put in a pot, cook on low heat and constantly stirring add 200mL of boiling water, then boil for another minute. Take 4-6 teaspoons after a meal every other day until the mixture is used up, then prepare the same amount and repeat the routine.

Note: If the diagnosis is the third or the fourth stage cancer that's spread to other parts of the body, and doctors don't give any chances for a cure, try the following.

Remedy #35
In a cup, mix 30mL unrefined sunflower oil or olive oil with 15mL spirit (96% proof). Put a lid on the cup, shake it for 2 minutes, and drink the mixture at once. Don't drink or eat anything else with it. Repeat this routine 3 times a day, 30 minutes before each meal. In case of nausea, chew on a piece of lemon peel and throw it away afterwards. Repeat this in three 10-day periods, always at the same times, taking a 5-day interval after each 10-day period. After the third cycle, take at least a 21-day interval before starting the next series. Don't use any other therapies during the interval; just allow your body to rest from the treatment.

While using this remedy, it's strictly prohibited to:

1. Use any other remedy, unless prescribed by medical doctor.
2. Interrupt the therapy before its completion
3. Reducing the dosage without consultation
4. Taking glucose intravenously
5. Drinking alcohol or smoking

Additional recommendations:

➢ Use only spirit that's at least 96% proof.
➢ The therapy can be started in any stage of the disease.
➢ Use only one kind of oil for the entire therapy.
➢ Eat according to guidelines (before remedy #34); don't use any other special diets or fasting routines.

> Cut your fat intake to a minimum.
> You can take painkillers that are not strong opiates. All other medications prescribed by your doctor can be taken, except hormonal formulas.

This therapy takes 3-4 months to cure stomach cancer in its first or second stage, 8-16 months for third or fourth stage cancer that's spread to other parts of the body. **Curing is impossible if the patient has used urine therapy. Urine therapy done without a complete body cleansing can be compared to suicide - it can cause cirrhosis of the liver in 3-4 months.**

In the first 4-10 days you may experience burning sensation and swelling in your throat. These discomforts will go away in 14-18 days.

Some food for thought

Cancer research involves a lot of scientists all over the world. Despite that, cancer is the cause of death in one of every three cases. The disease was first mentioned in some sources dated in the twelfth century BC. Serious research started in the nineteenth century AD. Today's classification contains over 150 kinds of cancers. There are many modern treatment methods utilizing the newest technology available today. Unfortunately, in too many cases oncologists remain helpless.

In "Hud-szi", an old Tibetan writing about curing diseases, the ancient doctors indicate that cancer is a specific kind of parasitic microorganism that poisons the host with its own toxic physiological products. The circulatory and skeletal systems are first to be affected, which results in aches and pains in joints, bones, and heart. Tibetan doctors called these parasites "white death". As time goes by, the parasites transform and grow into other parts of the body, forming tumors - "black death" or cancer.

Starting from this theory, biochemists from St. Petersburg tried to identify that parasite. Their research proved that cancer cells aren't mutated human cells, as is commonly believed, but Trichomonas, single-cell protozoan parasitic organisms living in all of us - one of the oldest on the planet. Research showed that Trichomonas have an amazing ability to transform and adapt to changing conditions - this is why they are so difficult to identify. For example, large doses of radiation, fatal for humans, have a stimulating effect on Trichomonas, causing even faster development and making them more "aggressive". Getting away from radiation, the parasites move from the tissue to blood and lymph, spreading that way in the entire body and starting to grow into new places. Perhaps this is why the most commonly used methods of treatment, such as chemotherapy and radiation, ease the symptoms temporarily but eventually intensify the disease. By analyzing records of patients that undergo those treatments, we can discover that most of them die within 3-10 years. Research also proved that when Trichomonas invade the tissues, they cause tumors, while their development in blood causes clots.

A hypothesis was put forward that AIDS virus is contained in these protozoan cells, not in lymphatic cells, as was commonly accepted. The fact that anti-virus medications are completely ineffective against AIDS supports this hypothesis. This means that our efforts against AIDS are going to be fruitless until we solve the cancer problem.

How do Trichomonas get into our body? Experiments done on animals and two-week-old embryos showed the presence of the parasites in the heart, brain, lungs, liver, kidneys, and large intestine. Cyst-like colonies have been found by dentists on their patients' gums. Women aged 16-58 taking part in the study had vaginal Trichomonas infections. Research done on a large population sample involving many professional backgrounds and an extensive geographical area proved that everybody is a carrier of the parasite. It lives in the mouth, the stomach area, and in the urogenital system. It can travel with blood and lymph to all organs in the body. The products of its physiology poison the host's nervous system, joints, liver, etc. This compromises the host's immunity, disrupts metabolism, and leads to countless health disorders.

Contemporary mainstream medicine doesn't recognize this theory as a valid one, even though there is no doubt about the soundness of science behind it. Three largest research institutes in Russia (Pasteur Epidemiology and Microbiology Institute, Rentgenology and Radiology Institute, and Otto Maternity and Gynecology Institute) confirmed all the facts in a five-year study. **Acceptance of this theory would mean a radical change in the established concepts of cancer treatment with all resulting expenditures of time, money, and other resources.**

I wouldn't like these facts to cause any panic in the reader. The theory states that we are all carriers of cancer cells, but how it practically plays out in our life depends on our immune system.

At the beginning of the twentieth century Dr. Passet proved that there are 23 kinds of bacteria in our brain tissue alone, among them staphylococci and tuberculosis bacteria. This doesn't necessarily mean that we have to go down with diseases caused by these bacteria. A healthy body has means of defending against thousands of diseases. There are many factors contributing to our health, such as hygiene, nutrition, or mental attitude. Until scientists and doctors discover the whole truth about cancer, people with even a slim chance for survival can take some steps to help themselves.

When analyzing cases of recovery from cancer in and outside of my own practice, I notice a certain pattern. People faced with the danger of death are usually motivated enough to radically change their lifestyle (body cleansing, proper nutrition, fasting, change of attitude and approach to problems, etc.), significantly build up their immunity, and conquer the disease as a result. Don't waste any more time. Start acting - it's all in your own hands.

What can we do to ensure a good chance of preventing cancers in our body? In one of my radio interviews, I answered this question the following way:

1. Eat fruits and vegetables grown in your geographical region and drink their freshly squeezed juices. There should be at least one apple and raw or cooked vegetables in your menu every day. Most valuable are vegetables and fruits with intensive green, orange, or red color (spinach, lettuce, cucumber, beans, peas, tomatoes, beets, carrot, pumpkin, pears, apples, etc.). They supply our body with all essential vitamins, minerals, fiber, and oxygen.

2. Know the difference among many kinds of fats. Fats are necessary for our body, especially at an advanced age. What kinds of fats are better? Plant oils, especially cold-pressed ones, contain acids and vitamins that extend our longevity. It is a good idea to take one teaspoon of oil every morning and evening and also to add one tablespoon of oil to your salads. The intake of meat, milk, and margarine should be limited.

3. Use more outdoor physical activity and learn to breathe correctly. Oxygen contained in the air is essential for each one of the billions of cells in our body and helps them regenerate, slowing down the aging process.

Physical activity allows oxygen to reach all cells - this is why it is better to exercise outdoors.

4. Be joyful! Your emotions affect not only your mind - they influence most physiological reactions in your body. When we are worried or irritated, our immune system (our body's natural defense system) stops issuing hormones T and B, which among others protect us from infections and cancer. When we are happy and enjoy our life, our immune system gets stronger and can better protect our health.

5. Find time to relax. Life in our modern world is full of tension and stress. They cannot be avoided but they should not be accumulated. Allow yourself time to do what you enjoy - go to your room and listen to favorite music, meditate, or take a walk in the woods. It helps to spend some time alone (3-5 minutes), relax, and forget all your troubles.

6. Keep your mind busy. The more your brain works the more stress it is able to bear. Regardless of your age, stimulate brain centers responsible for your memory. Read books, visit museums, listen to lectures, and play chess - in other words, use your head.

7. Get adequate amounts of sleep. Restful sleep clears the mind, relaxes muscles, reduces blood pressure, regenerates the hormonal system, and increases immunity. Even wounds heal better during sleep. People who are deprived of sleep for a few days show symptoms of psychological problems. Our demand for sleep varies. For some of us 4-5 hours is adequate while others need 8-10 hours. We should allow ourselves as much sleep as our body demands. This means that we should feel rested and refreshed when we get up.

8. Learn to enjoy walking. It is one of the ways to

keep your immune system strong. Maintaining the temperature in your bedroom at 61-63F (about16-17C) and taking alternate hot and cold showers every morning and evening also help develop your immunity.

9. Eat less; apply the principle of eating to live instead of living to eat. Chew your food slowly and leave the table while you still feel a slight sensation of hunger. Eat more natural products that do not undergo thermal processing (especially long frying).

10. Laugh more. Laughter engages more muscles than you realize. It massages our internal organs and stimulates the digestive system. It relieves pain and removes inflammations. We breathe deeper when we laugh, supplying more oxygen to our lungs. Our brain produces serotonin - the "happiness hormone." Finally, laughter often breaks the barriers in relations with other people.

11. Make love. Ancient medicine saw aspects of immortality in the union of male and female elements. The erotic act best rebuilds the harmony of our body.

12. Cleanse your body. Remember that its internal condition is going to be reflected in your external appearance.

13. Tune into what your body is telling you. The body can appreciate your concern. If you want to remain healthy, take care of yourself before the illness strikes.

Deadly radiation

Electromagnetic radiation has become a real hazard to our health. Its sources are everywhere. Can we keep ourselves safe from harmful rays? Yes, if we know and follow certain rules.

Why is electromagnetic radiation harmful?

The problem has been ignored by mainstream science until recently because it requires the acknowledgement of a controversial fact: human body has bio-poles. Only some physicists researched it, usually as a hobby.

It has been accurately determined now that each organ of our body works on a certain frequency: heart 700-800Hz, liver 300-400Hz, brain 10-15Hz (depending on the degree of stimulation). If our heart is exposed to radiation of similar frequency, it can increase or decrease the heart's frequency beyond the normal range. It can also happen with other organs. Exposure to electromagnetic fields of high intensity or even prolonged exposure to low intensity fields can lead to serious diseases.

Life on earth started and evolved in the environment with relatively weak electromagnetic radiation. Its sources were earth's own electromagnetic field, cosmic radiation, and solar radiation. Technical advances caused the total intensity of the field to increase a few units above those natural conditions. Our bio-poles (aura) are damaged mainly by above-ground power lines, radio communications, radio-location devices, and some other industrial infrastructure.

It has also been established that people living or working in the proximity of high-voltage power lines and sub-stations handling 500kW or more start feeling worse when the amount of power increases. The researchers found out that the odds of getting cancer increase several times for people living close to high-voltage power lines.

Health hazards in our own home

We might not even realize that we have many sources of harmful radiation in our home.

➤ Computer monitors and filters may be adequate to keep the user safe, but the radiation still doesn't disappear. It might concentrate at some point, e.g. a child's bed behind the operator's back. This is why it is important to position this modern device so that its radiation doesn't affect anybody and is aimed, for example, towards a window or a wall.

➤ Television should be watched from a distance of at least 2-3m. Not many people know that a TV set facing our bed can cause bone aches. Falling asleep with our TV on is even worse because in sleep our body is less able to protect against radiation. It's best to set a timer on our TV so that it turns itself off in case we fall asleep.

➤ Microwave ovens should have a built-in radiation-monitoring device. The oven's circuitry can get out of balance from time to time, causing a sharp increase in radiation intensity. A monitoring device alerts us when this happens, so that we can service the oven and bring everything back to normal.

Even common devices that are not as technological in nature, such as *lamps and chandeliers,* pose some degree of threat. The shape of chandeliers determines how radiation is directed. It's not a good idea to sit with a chandelier directly above our head. Our beds should be positioned in such a way that the head is not under a wall-mounted light. It's best to use half-spherical lights aimed at the ceiling.

It's better not to have a dresser in our bedroom. If there is one, make sure to have all mirrors lined in one plane, otherwise they can create zone with strong radiation. Mirrors mounted on the wall are in general much safer.

Architectural design of our home can have much to do with creating harmful radiation zones. The ideal shape for a room would be a round one. Since this is unrealistic, we can at least avoid sitting or lying down with our heads in the corner of a room - corners are the most dangerous places. It's not necessarily a superstition to avoid sitting at a table's corners - they act like antennas collecting radiation. Oval-shaped tables are much better.

As a general rule, it's a good idea to re-arrange furniture in our homes at least once a year in order to avoid constantly being exposed to the same pattern of radiation.

I've almost forgotten about one important device that's in common use these days - cellular telephones. Men often carry them in the inside pockets of their jackets, which causes prolonged exposure of their hearts and lungs to radiation. Keeping your telephone in a side-pocket, or even better, in your briefcase is much safer.

We can conclude that every contact with the environment influences our body's bi-poles to some degree. Even when we pull a blanket over ourselves, we can accept a 600-700V positive static charge. Walking on a synthetic carpet can charge us up to plus 1000V. Such influences cause accumulation of positive static electricity in our body, which is one of the causes of neural and cardiovascular disorders. Many scientists tend to believe that the excess of positive charges in our body can also be a factor in the formation of cancers.

We have all experienced small electrical discharges that sometimes happen when we shake hands with somebody or touch a grounded object. Nature provided a way for us to put our body's electric potential in balance by touching the ground with bare feet, which allows to accept negative electrical charge.

Charge up your body's battery

Unlike other mammals living on the Earth, humans walk on two legs. Our body acts like a battery with a positive charge in its upper parts including the head, and a negative charge in the lower body and legs. We get our positive charge from the universe and the negative one from the Earth. The higher the energy flow the healthier and more robust our body is. We acquire cosmic energy through breathing, contact with water (for example, when spending time at a lake or seashore), and eating plant-based foods. This is why we should maintain a close connection with air, water, and the world of plants. The charge from the Earth comes through our bare feet. Hippocrates wrote: **"Best footwear is no footwear."**

Our ancestors did not have fancy footwear with soles made of synthetic materials. They spent most of their lives barefoot and this is why they enjoyed better health and stronger immunity than we do today.

We live in very different circumstances created by our advanced civilization and spending much time barefoot is impossible. Some of the things we can do is walking barefoot on the morning dew, sandy beach, or snow for 1-2 minutes every day, or putting our feet under a stream of cold water. That way we build up our immunity against colds, flu, and many other health conditions.

Walking barefoot not only strengthens us and builds up our immunity but also prevents back, shoulder, and leg muscle pains. No matter what your age is, take therapeutic barefoot walks as often as possible. You will notice positive changes to your health from day to day: increased energy, better sleep, cheerful spirit, and a renewed zest for life.

Harmful radiation - the cause of many diseases

Only in theory our head has a positive and our legs a negative electrical charge. The balance is constantly being disturbed by a lot of small doses of radiation we absorb from our TV sets, computers, cars, clothing, etc. Following are a few simple methods to remove the effects of this radiation being one of the causes of various health disorders, and to restore your body's natural electrical balance.

Remedy #36

Take a flexible electrical wire which is not very thick (best copper) and remove the casing from both ends. Attach one end to something well-grounded a (e.g. plumbing or central heating installation). When planning to spend a longer period in one place (e.g. watching TV, reading, or just resting), wrap the other end of the wire around your wrist (left wrist is better - our hearts energy meridian runs that way). Remaining grounded that way for 2-3 hours will calm your nervous system and improve your sleep, making you more efficient at work and generally healthier.

Remedy #37

This method is not as effective, but it has an additional benefit of removing toxins from the body. Prepare a solution of salt (1g of salt per 1L of water) in a basin and put your feet in it, along with one end of your grounded wire. You can also put some pebbles or horse beans in the basin. Stepping on the pebbles or horse beans provides a foot massage, which helps in restoring your body's electrical balance.

Healing contact with trees

Contact with trees can also improve your electrical balance. Some trees can help you charge your body with beneficial energy while others make it possible to drain harmful energy. Both can be useful for fighting various health problems or generally improving our health.

Oak, pine, acacia, maple, rowan, birch, apple, cherry, plum, and pear trees are the ones bringing healthy energy into your body.

Remedy #38

To charge your body with healthy energy, stand 7-15inches (20-40cm) from a tree, facing away from it. Relax your muscles and close your eyes. Turn the palms of your hands towards the tree for 3-5 minutes and imagine how the tree's energy is flowing into you through your fingers.

Chestnut, poplar, willow, hazel, and aspen trees have the ability to drain harmful energy from your body.

Remedy #39

Face the tree from a distance of 7-12inches (20-30cm), turn the palms of your hands to the tree, and extend your arms towards it. Relax your muscles, close your eyes, and imagine the tree draining your body's unhealthy energy through the tips of your fingers. The session should last 10-15 minutes.

I have had a personal experience with the healing power of trees. I once had severe back pains and even painkillers could do nothing to ease the suffering. A few sessions with apple trees helped me to completely get rid of them.

Contemporary people who are used to rely on modern science may have hard time accepting the fact that contact with and ordinary tree can remedy a health problem better than our sophisticated medical science. There are many mysteries in nature. We should accept and make use of undeniable facts even if we don't have any explanation for them.

Combing hair with a wooden comb was an ancient remedy against insomnia and nervous exhaustion. Siberian healers told their patients to hold a chunk of aspen wood in their mouths for relief against strong toothaches. Pieces of birch wood were used to heal many feminine disorders and hemorrhoids. Putting chunks of aspen against certain spots on the head helped against schizophrenia, epilepsy, and headaches.

Ending this incomplete description of the healing power of trees, I'd like to mention another interesting remedy. It deals with staphylococcus aureus - an infection which is pretty hard to defeat even with today's medicinal formulas. I've had a few patients with staphylococcus aureus infections in the eyes, throat, and nose. They suffered a lot of pain. Antibiotics and other expensive medications couldn't bring any relief - the bacteria seemed to be immune to everything. My remedy surprised them at first. However, when they tried it out they learned that simple-sounding solutions can sometimes be the most brilliant ones.

Remedy #40 (against staphylococcus aureus infections)
Use a few birch logs (preferably soaked by rainwater) to make a fire. Sit by the fire and allow smoke to get into your respiratory passages and your eyes. It will cause some discomfort - you have to suffer through it. To ease eye itching, you can rub the eyes with your hands. It strengthens the therapeutic effect because there is some residue on your

hands from handling the birch logs. The next day you should be free of any symptoms of infection. If it doesn't work the first time, repeat the routine.

Other Health Issues

When modern medicine writes off a disease as incurable, the only remaining solution is to turn for help to the Mother Nature.

Some remarks about diabetes

Thirty or forty years ago, when we didn't have today's abundance of highly processed refined food, deli products, baked goods containing white refined flour, sweets, and sweet beverages, diabetes was a rare disease. People who got it were usually advanced in years and their pancreas wasn't efficient any longer due to old age.

Today, diabetes cases can be found in younger generation, even among children. The main cause of the disease, no matter the age, is our diet, rich in fried or cooked meat, sweet baked goods, and pasteurized or cooked cow milk.

Taking insulin isn't effective in curing diabetes. Insulin is a hormone produced by pancreas and it allows the body to assimilate natural organic sugars. The energy acquired that way is used in metabolic processes and for the nourishment and regeneration of pancreas itself. Our cells can use natural organic sugars found in large amounts in fruits and vegetables, but not

manufactured sugars or starch found in fries, white-flour baked goods, or overcooked grains. These harmful products still
have to be processed by our body. They first have to be broken
down into simple sugars. Thermal processing destroys all active enzymes in those foods (the enzymes break down in temperatures above 130F (54C), so our body has to use more of its
own resources. This way our pancreas becomes overworked
because the demand for insulin is much higher than its normal
output. On top of that, the products of such digestion are non-
organic atoms substances that can't be used for regenerating
the pancreas, and this leads to diabetes. Insulin shots can be
compared to loans we take when we spend money faster than
we can earn it. Borrowing involves costs. In case of insulin
shots, the price we pay is cardiovascular disorders, gallbladder
stones, and kidney stones.

Most people with diabetes are overweight. This is because
synthetic, industrially produced insulin promotes fat accumulation rather than its burning. Accumulated fats and toxins cause
circulatory disorders. The blood becomes thick and acidic,
which leads to heart disorders and calcium stones.

Diabetes is frequently the result of a strong psychological
stress. It usually happens in people whose liver is weak or who
suffer from large intestine disorders. Stress usually affects our
liver, which is our body's "chemical laboratory." A malfunctioning liver causes disorders in other organs cooperating with
it, the digestive system and pancreas. This can lead to ulceration of the stomach or duodenum or to diabetes. People with
diabetes who don't get insulin shots have a better chance against the disease. Most of my patients, especially those who
didn't take insulin, were completely cured.

We know that our digestive system, if fed natural non-pro-
cessed food, can produce all hormones necessary for our body,
including insulin. It means that we can get rid of diabetes by

putting some effort into changing our diet. What steps should we undertake? First, exclude or minimize the amount thermally processed products containing concentrated starch and sugars, such as bread, peeled and boiled potatoes, refined sugar and products containing it (e.g. commercially available fruit juices), overcooked grains, cooked meat, pasteurized or cooked milk and its products (commercial yogurt, kefir, cheese, and butter). Eat only homemade cheeses, butter, and yogurts. Prepare your own cereals to make sure they are not overcooked. You need to eat grains everyday. The healthiest types of grains are buckwheat, wheat, corn, barley, and rice (especially wild, unrefined). It is better to cook grains with small amounts of water. One third of our diet should consist of grains. When cooking grains it is best to use the interrupted cooking method. For example, buckwheat can be prepared in the following way:

1. Rinse the buckwheat and soak it for 3-4 hours
2. Do not change the water; cook buckwheat for 3-5 minutes
3. Cut some onion into small pieces; add it to the pot
4. Wrap the pot in a towel to maintain the temperature for 15-30 minutes
5. Add some cold-pressed vegetable oil before eating.

The main part of your diet should be fresh or dried fruits and vegetables, freshly squeezed fruit and vegetable juices, other dishes based on fruits and vegetables (best baked in the oven), grains, some nuts, and honey in place of sugar. For fats use only cold-pressed vegetable oils. It's beneficial to drink 1qt (1L) of the following juice mixtures every day: 12oz (360g) carrot, 8oz (240g) lettuce, 180g bean sprouts, and 6oz (180g) cabbage (proportion 6:4:3:3), plus half a liter of juice mixture made of 9.3oz (280g) carrot and 4oz (120g) spinach. The result of your therapy will be even better if you cleanse your large intestine using an enema and go through a liver cleansing procedure every three months. (See "Can We Live 150 Years? p. 189-198).

I would like to treat the subject of enema (intestinal irrigation) in more detail because enema is one of the most effective procedures you can do at home to clean toxins from your body.

Some specialists warn that large intestine irrigation destroys the healthy microflora. I do not agree with that. It is almost impossible to find a person with a healthy microflora because of our diet, lack of exercise, and the amount of medications (especially antibiotics) we take. I would guess that about 90% of people have a degenerated digestive tract and a damaged microflora. Dr. Norman Walker, an American physician known around the world (he lived for 106 years) used enema for 50 years to treat different diseases. He regarded enema to be the simplest and most effective method to clean internal filth from the body. He used to say that people who do not believe in enema's effectiveness need it most.

Practice shows that many people are not ready to use the large intestine irrigation routine because it seems repulsive to them. They should realize that it is the only way to remove layers of stagnant fecal matter accumulated in their intestine. Stagnant matter looks much more repulsive, and its smell is worse than the worst sewage system smell you can imagine. Other people find the position inconvenient or do not have enough space at home to perform the procedure. There are many excuses. But the threat of an operation or death provides an instant motivation to try putting their large intestine in order. The most reasonable behavior is to start using the procedure before we are faced with any serious health threats.

Before I start describing the procedure in detail, I would like you to remember two things. First, your motivation can be provided by the desire to get rid of stagnant deposits that cause many health problems. Second, you must follow the prescribed routine in detail to avoid harming yourself and to achieve maximum benefits.

The technique of enema - large intestine irrigation

Make a solution of 1.5-2 quarts (1.5-2L) of boiled water (at body temperature) and 1-2 tablespoons of lemon juice (filter pulp and seeds out of the juice). Put the solution in the enema bag (available in most pharmacies).

Hang the bag about 3-5ft (1-1.5m) above your body level; apply some vegetable oil to the enema tubing and your anus. Vegetable oil is preferred to vaseline, creams, or soap because it is a natural product and does not plug up skin pores. Assume the "tiger position" - down on your knees and elbows, your legs slightly spread, your abdomen relaxed as much as possible. Insert the end of the tubing into your anus and let water flow into it. Breathe deeply through the open mouth. The enema bag will be empty in 1-2 minutes and then you can get up. (If water does not flow freely from the bag, squeeze the enema tube to stop the flow completely for a few seconds and then let the water flow again.)

This is not the end of the procedure. You should shake up your intestine a little. One of the ways to do it is to do some jumping and shaking of the lower abdomen with your hands. In any way, try to create some washing action inside your intestine, then lie on your back and wait. You will feel a bowel movement reflex in 2-10 minutes. Be prepared to spend 15-20 minutes on the toilet - take a magazine or a book to read. Eventually you will feel that all water has left your large intestine (urination is the final sign).

If you are new to the procedure, it is a good idea to take a look at the waste washed out with water. The sight is unpleasant, even repulsive, but this is what it takes to provide strong motivation for the future.

The routine should be repeated every day in the first week, every second day in the second and third week, and twice in the fourth week.

After the fourth week, most of you will know by the look and smell of your stools that the cleaning has been successful. To maintain your large intestine in this clean state from then on, it is enough to perform the routine once a week for the rest of your life.

What you have just done can be compared to cleaning up soil around your body's "roots" by removing layers of hardened fecal matter, mold, putrefaction and fermentation products. Now these roots can absorb useful substances from the digested food, needed to build new cells. Your body absorbs no more harmful and carcinogenic toxins. Now your blood can be cleansed and the development of diseases reversed. You have achieved it all by yourself.

All organs can receive better nutrition, and clean blood is able to dissolve harmful deposits in other parts of the body. Internal organs gradually return to their proper places, their functioning improves, blood pressure normalizes from day to day, and no diseases affect your body anymore.

Our large intestine that has been stretched, withered, and malnourished for a long time has to be returned to its proper shape in order to efficiently perform its important functions. When it is returned to the natural shape, it learns again to move along the masses of undigested food and other waste.

In order to achieve this, we can eat a lot of grains during the weeks of our enema therapy (it is a good idea at any time). Make sure it is whole grains. Use only water to prepare them. As a grain meal passes through the stomach, small intestine, and then enters the large intestine, it helps the large intestine assume the proper shape. **NOTE:** Just remember not to use any milk in preparing your grains.

I presented Dr. Walker's intestinal irrigation as the simplest and most effective method of cleaning up layers of hardened feces from your large intestine. Some people can't accept this method and try other ways to achieve intestinal cleansing.

Many ill people still fear the irrigation procedure and want to use laxatives for intestinal cleansing. I definitely discourage the use of laxatives. They dry up the intestines and cause dehydration of our entire body. Our large intestine's muscles should be made to work. Laxatives cause the emptying of the intestine without engaging the muscle tissue, which leads to its weakening. Weak intestinal muscles, in turn, cause chronic constipation. Enema, in contrast, stimulates and normalizes our large intestine's function. People who went through a series of enemas do not suffer from constipation.

To bring the expected results, all cleansing routines have to be done in the appropriate order. You just learned about the first step - large intestine cleansing. There is no other way to start complete body cleansing. If you try to skip it and go ahead with the other routines, they will not produce results.

This may be better understood in the context of another secret to maintaining good health: For best results, internal hygiene must go together with smart nutrition. You will be fully protected from any diseases by applying this principle. Intestinal cleaning itself does not protect us from huge energy losses in the process of digesting improperly combined meals. Similarly, a proper diet will not stop deadly toxins accumulated in our large intestine from being absorbed in the blood stream. On the contrary, it stimulates the absorbing functions. There is only one way to go - cleansing has to be done by performing the whole presented set of routines.

In addition to these recommendations, some remedies are listed below for you to try as a supplementary measure against diabetes. By watching their effects on your health and overall mood, you can select one that works best for you.

Remedy #41

Ingredients: 3.5oz (100g) of onion juice and 3.5oz (100g) of honey

Preparation: Peel 1 onion, grate it finely, squeeze the juice into a jar, add honey, mix well, close tightly, and store in a dark place.

Usage: Take 2 teaspoons 3 times a day before meals for one month.

Remedy #42

Ingredients: 0.35oz (10g) of unripe green walnuts (harvested before Jul 7)

Preparation: Chop the walnuts finely, put them in a cup, fill with boiling water, and cover with a lid for 15 minutes.

Usage: Drink warm like a tea.

Remedy #43

Ingredients: 3 cups of ripe oats

Preparation: Put the oats in an enamel pot and pour 600mL of boiling water on it. Put a lid on it and warm up for 15 minutes, stirring from time to time, then let it cool at room temperature for 45 minutes. Strain the brew into a glass bottle, squeezing all liquid out of the oats, then add some boiled water to have full 600mL of liquid, and close with a cork. Store in a cool place for 2 days at most.

Usage: Drink half a cup of warm liquid 3-4 times a day before meals. The therapy lasts 3 months.

Remedy #44
Ingredients: 10 average-sized bay leaves
Preparation: Break up the leaves, put in a glass or enamel vessel, pour 600mL (about 3 cups) of boiling water over them, cover with a lid, and let it stand for 2-3 hours.
Usage: Drink half a cup of warm formula 3-4 times a day for two weeks, take a one-month interval, and then repeat the therapy.

Remedy #45
Ingredients: Sweet potato leaves (2oz /60g fresh or 1oz / 30g dried), white pumpkin peel (3.3oz /100g fresh or 0.4oz /12g dried)
Preparation: Chop finely and cook.
Usage: Drink like a tea at any time of the day.

Remedy #46
Ingredients: 15 dried plums
Preparation: Put in a pot with boiling water and boil for a while.
Usage: Drink warm, like a tea.

Remedy #47
Ingredients: 50 green pea pods
Preparation: Cook for 20 minutes.
Usage: Drink the brew and eat the pods once a day.

Viva potatoes

I'm going to explain a few things about important benefits and potential dangers of eating potatoes, a valuable and easily available gift from nature. First, I'd like to tell the story of Alma Niekse, a girl living in Copenhagen some years ago, who overcame an incurable debilitating disease using ordinary potatoes. Life treated her harshly from childhood - she had polyarthritis, deforming her body. Her posture was twisted, joints swollen, and fingers curved. Her mother was the only support she had during twenty years spent in a wheelchair. When her mother died, the girl spent sleepless nights alone with her desperation, often contemplating suicide. Suddenly one night she had an unexpected revelation showing her a way to become healthy. She couldn't rationally explain how it happened. It was almost as if her guardian angel whispered to her, "If you want to get well, boil potatoes with peels for a long time, make a pulp of them, and eat nothing but that pulp all day long." After two weeks of following this advice, the girl noticed some improvement. Her teeth weren't as clenched, she could open her mouth easier, and the joints didn't hurt as much as before. A month's time brought even more change - she seemed to be a different person. She ate exclusively potato pulp for a total of three months, which completely returned her to health.

Many readers are going to just smile at this incredible-sounding story. How can somebody miraculously receive exact instructions for a cure? Whether we believe in miracles or not, we know that there are a lot of undiscovered intuitive abilities in our mind. All of us have intuitive insights. I use intuition a lot in advising my patients and, as a rule, they are not disappointed.

Going back to Alma's story, when she got well, she wanted to help other people with similar conditions. She went to hospitals and doctors' offices, telling everybody about a simple way to treat polyarthritis. Nobody wanted to believe her, but she didn't quit. She went on to study medicine and become a physician, using both her knowledge and experience for helping people. Today, in her eighties, she is still healthy and physically fit.

Why aren't potatoes appreciated today as much as they deserve to be? It's because we want to be smarter than nature. In the old days, they were considered as important as bread. Our grandmothers always boiled or roasted them complete with the peels and served them as a separate dish, with sauerkraut or cucumber. Nobody thought of peeling potatoes and cutting them into fries. Such fries cause nothing but fat tissue and constipation. We misuse potatoes in the same way we misuse sugar beets by taking a valuable nutritious product and making it into a poison in the form of whit refined sugar. It's the same case with white flour - we throw away the grain's vitamin-rich enclosure and keep white poisonous starch. Complete potatoes with peels contain much more than starch. There are also enzymes, proteins, vitamins B and C, beta carotene, organic acids, mineral salts, potassium, calcium, phosphorus, iron, and many other useful substances. Up to 90% of them are found in the peel. According to the newest research, substances found in potato peel have medicinal properties helpful against allergies, high blood pressure, arrhythmia, diabetes, stomach ulceration, and inflammations of the liver, bile ducts, or kidneys. These substances participate in many organic processes happening in the body. They help strengthen the walls of our blood vessels. It's still an incomplete list of their health benefits. This is why we should be skeptical about recipes that tell us to use peeled potatoes. Enzymes found in complete potatoes transform starch into easily assimilated sugars that are a source of energy, and the by-products of the reaction are removed from the body.

Starch by itself isn't water-soluble. Glue-like chunks of starch can plug up blood vessels, causing arteriosclerosis and other damage. Cooked starch is poor in oxygen, which prevents its full burning, which leads to fat tissue formation. Excessive consumption of fries in the 1980-ties caused obesity and many other disorders in the American population. Many Americans suffer from health problems today as a result of their liking for fries.

I will repeat for the benefit of those who enjoy eating potatoes: peeling robs potatoes of practically 99% of valuable compounds. Some people don't like the way potato peel tastes and smells, but much depends on the way we prepare our potatoes. You can put your potatoes into boiling water and add some herbs and other spices, to improve the taste. It's even healthier to steam potatoes. I usually wash potatoes, cut them in halves, put in the oven, put some cumin, marjoram, and other spices on them, and then bake for 40-45 minutes. They can be served with some butter, chopped parsley, dill, or chive. It's a very healthy meal, especially in combination with cabbage, cucumbers, or sour milk.

Some people peel vegetables to remove toxic chemicals. Recent studies prove that high content of iron in the peels of carrots, beets, potatoes, and apples prevent accumulation of toxins. I advise to give up potatoes in the spring time, starting about March 1, because that's when their vegetation period starts and a toxic substance is produced that can cause weakness, sleepiness, and headaches.

We should be aware that some potatoes are treated with Cesium-137 and Cobalt-60 radiation for storage. It gives them longer shelf life and attractive appearance, but carries a risk of causing cancer in people who eat them.

Now that we know about the health benefits and potential dangers of eating potatoes, I'll give two more simple recipes.

1. Boiled potatoes with cumin

Wash and boil whole potatoes, then carefully take off the very outside layer of the peel. Put some vegetable oil, cumin, and chopped parsley or dill on them.

2. Potatoes with mushrooms.

Steam your potatoes and take off the very outside layer of the peel. Cook some mushrooms separately in a small amount of water, chop them finely, and put on top of the potatoes. Add some onion (fried on vegetable oil) and chopped parsley or dill.

Healing power of apples

We all know the saying, "One apple a day keeps the doctors away." An entire book could be dedicated to the health benefits of eating apples. There are plenty of sources that describe substances found in apples, such as vitamins and organic acids. I'm going to mention here a few remedies that use the healing power of apples. Apple juice works wonders at cleansing our body, especially liver, kidneys, and gallbladder.

Liver cleansing with apple juice

Use only freshly squeezed juice (store bought juices do not bring the expected results). Use mostly sweet apples - add just a few from a sour variety to achieve a pleasant taste. Drink in small sips and hold each sip in your mouth for a while to let it blend with your saliva. People with unhealthy digestive tract micro-flora can suffer from some stomach discomfort, such as bloat-ing, after drinking the juice. To prevent the discomfort, they can filter the remaining pulp particles from the juice. You can earlier prepare your digestive system to be able to handle high acid content by drinking half a glass of apple juice 15 minutes before every meal during the proceeding week. The cleansing lasts three days. You have to abstain from any food. Outdoor physical activity would be beneficial.

Each day of the procedure, drink only apple juice in the fol-lowing amounts:

8 a.m.	- 1 glass
10 a.m.	- 1 glass
12 noon	- 2 glasses
2 p.m.	- 2 glasses
4 p.m.	- 2 glasses
6 p.m.	- 1 glass
8 p.m.	- 1 glass

If there is no bowel movement during the therapy, you can drink stool-stimulating herbal beverages or, even better, per-form an enema.

Apple cider vinegar

Many people use large amounts of vinegar for seasoning or in preparation of food products. Wine vinegar and white distilled vinegar contain ingredients that harm our health, for example acetic acid ($C_2H_4O_2$). Acetic acid destroys red blood cells, causes anemia, interferes with the digestive processes, and impedes food absorption. It causes cirrhosis (a chronic liver disease), ulcerative inflammations of the large intestine, etc. (beware if you like pickled cucumbers and mushrooms or different pickled salads). My advice is not to use spirit vinegar if you want to avoid digestive tract problems.

Apple vinegar has entirely different qualities. It contains malic acid ($C_4H_6O_5$). When it reacts with bases and minerals, it produces glycogen, which helps regulate the menstrual cycle, improves the condition of blood vessels, and promotes the building of red blood cells. One of the most valuable qualities of apple vinegar is very high content of potassium, necessary for calming the nervous system, regulating the hormonal function, and retaining calcium, iron, magnesium, and silicon in our body. Apple vinegar can be bought in stores or prepared at home.

Apple cider vinegar therapies

Shingles
Apply a gauze pad soaked in undiluted apple cider vinegar on the affected areas 4 times during the day and 3 times at night (if itching does not let you sleep). The remedy relieves the pain in 5-10 minutes and cures shingles in 3-7 days.

Night sweating
Rub apple vinegar on your skin before bedtime.

Burns
Use a gauze pad soaked in apple cider vinegar to wash the affected areas. It relieves pain and prevents scarring.

Varicose veins

Wash the skin in the area of dilated veins with a pad soaked in apple cider vinegar in the morning and in the evening. In addition, drink a solution of 2 teaspoons of apple cider vinegar in a cup of warm boiled water twice a day. The dilated veins usually start narrowing after a month of regular therapy.

Weight reduction therapy

Drink a cup of boiled water with 2 teaspoons of apple cider vinegar before every meal.

Excessive secretion of tears

Make a solution of 1 teaspoon of apple cider vinegar and 1 drop of iodine in 1 cup of water. Drink every day for 2 weeks; then drink twice a week (e.g. Tuesday and Thursday) for two months.

Limping caused by joint inflammation

Take 10 teaspoons of apple cider vinegar before every meal. The therapy should reduce pain in 20% after 2 days, 50% after 5 days, and remove the pain completely after 30 days.

High blood pressure

Some people have high blood pressure caused by a deficiency of hydrochloric acid in their digestive tract. It is necessary to lower the intake of meat to effectively treat this condition. A noticeable reduction of blood pressure can be achieved by taking 1 to 3 teaspoons of apple cider vinegar before every meal. For better effects, you can occasionally take apple cider vinegar with a teaspoon of honey.

Headaches

Pour half a cup of apple cider vinegar and half a cup of boiled water in a pot. Mix the solution, heat up slowly to the point of boiling, and turn off the heat. Slowly inhale the vapor 75 times. The headache will be removed or at least significantly reduced.

Making apple cider vinegar

The amount of ingredients depends on the amount of apple cider vinegar you need for your specific use. Cut out rotten and damaged parts of the apples. Grind or crush the apples (including the peel and seeds with their enclosures). Put the pulp in an enamel or glass container with a wide opening and add warm boiled water (1 quart/1L of water per 28oz/800g of apple pulp). Add 3.5oz (100g) of honey, 0.35oz (10g) of baker's yeast, and 0.7oz (20g) of dried dark bread per 1 quart (1L) of water. Cover the container with a lid and let it stand in the temperature of 68-86F (20-30C) for fermentation (steady temperature and wide container opening improve fermentation). Stir it with a wooden spoon every day.

After ten days, put it in a gauze bag and squeeze juice from it. Filter the juice into a container with a wide opening. Add 2.8oz (80g) of honey per 1 quart (1L) of juice and stir until honey is dissolved. Cover the container with a gauze pad and let it stand in the temperature of 77-86F (25-30C). The vinegar is ready when its color turns light. It usually takes 40-60 days, depending on the kind of apples, honey, the amount of water, and some other factors. When the fluid turns light, use a funnel to pour it into half-liter bottles, close the bottles tightly with a cork stopper (you can pour some wax on top of the stopper to close it more tightly), and store in a cool place. You can use it as a remedy (see the section below) or as seasoning with your salads and other food. I would like to stress again, that apple cider vinegar is the only acidic seasoning to be used with your food.

When you catch a cold

In spring and fall, we often catch cold or flu, starting with a runny nose, headaches, and general body weakness. It can be looked at as our body's defense mechanisms in action: mucus is eliminated through every possible outlet, carrying away disease-causing bacteria we allowed to breed in our body through excessive consumption of meat, fats, sweets, and other unhealthy foods. Our body tries to clean itself. This defensive reaction is sometimes accompanied by higher body temperature. If the fever doesn't get too high, we shouldn't hurry in applying anti-fever medication. It's better to wait the usual 4-7 days and allow the process to run its course. You can help along by applying the following advice:

1. In the first two days, give up all food except fruits and vegetables and their freshly squeezed juices, or go through a body detoxification routine (page 49).
2. Drink a lot (1-3qt /1-3L a day) of warm beverages brewed from currants, raspberry, or wild blueberry with some honey. This helps mucus to get released from our body and carry away toxins.
3. Air your home regularly - high oxygen content speeds up your body's cleansing process.
4. Take an alternate hot and lukewarm shower for 2-3 minutes 4 times a day. It provides a hydro-massage for your blood vessels, helping them to clean.
5. After the massage, soak a small towel in a solution of regular

table salt (4 tablespoons of salt in a liter of water) and rub your entire body with it. Put fresh clothes on your moist body.

6. A helpful method to overcome any infection is garlic enema. It should be done in the morning and evening in the first three days. Add juice squeezed from one half of a garlic clove to 200mL of warm boiled water. Put some vegetable oil on the end of enema tubing and the opening of your rectum and proceed as in a regular enema. An additional benefit from this procedure is an improvement of your skin complexion.

7. Don't be too quick in deciding to take temperature-reducing medication and antibiotics. They interfere with your body's natural defense mechanisms. Even though they destroy some disease-causing bacteria, they do even more damage to your useful microflora. Disease causing bacteria are going to attack you again sooner or later. Damage done to your intestinal tract's natural microflora takes a long time to be repaired. Folk medicine has a safer way of dealing with fever. Add 5 tablespoons of apple cider vinegar to 1qt (1L) of warm water. Using a sponge, apply the solution on your entire body, and without toweling, put your clothes on. Take an alternate shower after 30-40 minutes. If this doesn't work, soak a pair of thin cotton socks in apple cider vinegar or wine vinegar, put them on, and put a pair of thick warm socks on top of them. Go to bed, cover yourself well, and drink enough raspberry tea with honey to stimulate heavy sweating.

Raspberries instead of aspirin pills

Raspberries contain acetylsalicylic acid (ASA), or aspirin, in its natural organic form that doesn't cause any side effects.

Experienced physicians always warn their patients not to overuse aspirin pills because it causes damage to intestinal tract's mucous membrane. Many ill people don't tolerate aspirin pills. They can use raspberries instead, which among other benefits would have a soothing effect on their stomach.

Researchers from the state of Michigan discovered that aspirin prevents the formation of malignant tumors and can neutralize the carcinogenic effect of nicotine. According to the study, the risk of cancer could be significantly reduced by taking 2-3 aspirin pills a day. This became a worldwide news story and aspirin sales grew rapidly. At about the same time, other researchers in the state of Vermont made another discovery that had no apparent connection with aspirin. They found that some kinds of progressive degenerative diseases (including Parkinson's and Alzheimer's diseases) are caused by high levels of aluminum in the body. Alzheimer's disease, a particularly severe form of progressive impairment, affected almost three million Americans. What does it have to do with aspirin? Aluminum is one of the components of synthetic aspirin pills of various brands. While helping us deal with one health issue, these pills create another problem. **The use of aluminum pots, food wrappers, and beverage cans also contributes to high levels of aluminum in our body.**

Nature gives us in raspberries not only aspirin but also vitamins A, B, C, K, and E. Many other useful ingredients (e.g. mineral salts of iron, calcium, and potassium) help improve blood circulation, cleanse blood, heal swellings, and reduce headaches. There are among them good antiseptics, painkillers, and other substances inducing sweat or urination, building up immunity, and preventing cancer. Most important, they don't cause any side effects.

All described medicinal properties are found not only in the fruit, but also in raspberry leaves and twigs. Medicinal raspberry beverage can be prepared the following way:

Remedy #48

Ingredients: 1 tablespoon of raspberry fruits (fresh or dried), chopped leaves, or twigs

Preparation: Pour 1 cup of boiling water on the fruits, leaves, or twigs, let it stand for 20 minutes and add 1 teaspoon of honey.

Usage: Drink the beverage, and then lie in bed warmly covered for a while. Repeat 4-5 times a day. Drink it warm while you are still down with a cold or flu. When you start getting over the disease, you can drink it at any temperature.

Eating raspberries has great benefits but, as in everything else, moderation is important. Don't eat more than 4-5 tablespoons a day. You don't need too much of a good thing.

Raspberry elixir

Ingredients: 4 tablespoons of raspberry juice, lemon juice (from half a lemon), 2 cups of water, 2 tablespoons of honey

Preparation: Blend the ingredients and add 2 ice cubes.

Raspberry kefir

Ingredients: 8 tablespoons of stirred fresh raspberries, 1 cup of kefir (sour milk would be even better), some honey

Preparation: Blend the ingredients.

Raspberry-gooseberry cocktail
   Ingredients: 5.3oz (150g) of raspberries, 5.3oz (150g) of gooseberries, 1 cup of mineral water, 2 tablespoons of honey
   Preparation: Squeeze the fruits and strain juice out, then add water and honey to it.

Some remedies suggested in this book may require more time and diligence than readers can afford in our busy times. Folk medicine knows many simple remedies that don't take any effort at all. For example, when you first start feeling like you are catching a cold, try a preventative measure that's been used by Siberian people for centuries. They put a pebble in their mouth and suck on it like on a candy. This is related to children's thumb-sucking reflex, which is a way of building up immunity against infections. Doctors call this method self-deceptive, but some studies suggest a good explanation of the mechanism. Sucking on a pebble stimulates heavy salivation, and this in turn helps dissolve immunity-building minerals contained in the pebble. Intensive blood circulation through the mouth (about 4L in half an hour) distributes dissolved substances throughout the body. We can only admire the wisdom of our ancestors, who passed down to us a remedy that's simple, effective, and available without prescription. If you don't have a pebble handy or worry about accidentally swallowing it, you can suck on raisins or apricots, the result will be just as good.

Prevent food poisoning

Even a tidy-looking kitchen may not be free of health hazards. The biggest danger comes from bacteria that can cause food poisoning. It doesn't have to manifest itself through vomiting, abdominal pains, or dizziness. Symptoms may be as mild as a slight headache, sleepiness, or the feeling of weakness. We wouldn't usually associate such symptoms with a warmed up meal we've just had that we cooked the previous evening and left at room temperature overnight. In order to minimize the danger of food poisoning, use the following rules in your kitchen.

1. Don't leave any food (including vegetables and baked goods) non-refrigerated for longer than 1.5 hours. Bacteria can quickly multiply even at room temperature.
2. Have at least four cutting boards, separate for fruits and vegetables, meat, fish, and deli products. Plastic boards are the most practical because they are easy to wash and don't retain smells. After preparing your meals, thoroughly clean and disinfect your kitchen table, sink, and all accessories.
3. Wash your eggs before cooking them.

If you happen to get food poisoning, try one of these two remedies:

Remedy #49
Pour a cup of boiling water on 1 teaspoon of tea (preferably green), let it stand for 5-10 minutes, then add 2 tablespoons of milk (or 3 teaspoons of coffee cream) and 1 teaspoon of salt. Stir the mixture well and drink it. This will cleanse your digestive tract and prevent it from forming gases.

Remedy #50
Take half a cup of well-rinsed raisins, pour boiling water on them to fill the cup, let the brew stand until it cools down, and than drink it. The remedy cleans your tongue and intes-

tines, heals intestinal inflammations, and removes constipation.

Tea can be also used as an antidote in cases of alcohol poisoning (hangover). Moderate consumption of alcohol isn't harmful in itself, it can even be beneficial. This is especially true if it's shared with a group of friends in a relaxing atmosphere that includes social chat and a lot of laughter. Drinking 25-50ml of liquor or 100-150ml of good red wine a day not only relaxes your nervous system but also prevents heart disease and circulatory system problems. Some studies suggest that it can lower the risk of heart attack by as much as 40%, which is consistent with my own observations.

Some people take 1-2 tablespoons of vodka or brandy before going to bed in order to improve their sleep. They say it also improves their memory, appetite, and overall mood. Hippocrates said that the same substance can be a poison or a remedy, depending on the dose. It's good to keep this in mind when we drink so that we don't have to deal with a hangover the next day.

Remedy #51

Hot, strong, and sweet tea with milk or cream is a good antidote against alcohol poisoning (hangover) or medication overdose. Simply pour 100ml of boiling water on 1 teaspoon of green or black tea, add 4 teaspoons of sugar and 2 tablespoons of milk or 2 teaspoons of coffee cream.

What about a cup of tea

There are two schools of thought about the effects of drinking tea. Some believe that drinking tea is necessary to maintain good functioning of the heart and blood vessels, and they recommend 5-6 cups a day. Others advise to avoid tea altogether as the main factor damaging our digestive tract, increasing the acidity of our blood, and harming our general health. As usual, the truth is in the middle. We can and should drink tea, provided it is fresh and correctly prepared. Fresh tea (not older than 1 hour) expands our blood vessels, improves our heart function, rejuvenates the nervous system, removes fatigue, cleanses blood, helps eliminate radioactive elements, gives some relief against migraine headaches, and has cancer-preventing properties. Such tea contains about 80 medicinal substances, catechins being the most important of them.

Rinse a porcelain teapot with boiling water, put 1 teaspoon of tea and 1 teaspoon of sugar in it, and pour 1 cup of boiling water on them. Put the lid on the pot and cover it with a towel for 5-10 minutes. Drinking 2-3 such servings a day is beneficial to your health.

Every positive change we experience contributes to a more hopeful outlook on life.

Kiss Baldness Goodbye

For some men, the thought of getting bold is scarier than the thought of becoming impotent. The fear of balding is surprisingly strong, probably because we subconsciously associate our hair's thickness with good level of sexual performance. And while impotence can be kept secret, baldness is rather difficult to hide.

Historians say that Julius Caesar liked to wear his laurel wreath on all occasions mainly because it efficiently concealed the bold spot on his head. And when Napoleon Bonaparte met with the Russian emperor Alexander to discuss the future of Europe, the meeting ended with a chat about anti-balding formulas. Most balding men are willing to try any medication that gives them even a glimpse of hope. People, who otherwise have a lot of common sense and life experience, can be fooled into relying on vague promises and absurd-sounding methods.

For centuries, dishonest dealers built their fortunes by selling "miraculous" cures to the afflicted men, who never gave up their hope for a miracle. I don't like having to disappoint them, but in fact there are no miracles in this case. The closest we can get is by trying to learn about and deal with the real causes of hair loss.

The topic is particularly close to my heart because I've been working for years, day after day, in order to hold on to every hair still remaining on my own head. I can boast some measure of success - there hasn't been any hair loss in the last few years, there even seems to have been some re-growth. Many of those who have used my advice have better reasons to show off their re-grown hair than I do. As is often the case, it turns out that the physician cannot cure himself.

Let's take a look at the phenomenon. A human scalp sheds about 50-100 hairs a day. We find them on our comb, brush, pillow, etc. This is no reason to worry because this kind of shedding is part of a natural cycle. Every hair remains on our scalp for an average of four years, growing at the rate of 1-1.5cm a month, and then "retires" for about three months and is replaced by a new hair.

The mechanics of balding

Our scalp has the most elaborate network of blood vessels and needs higher blood supply compared to other parts of our body. At the base of each hair, there is the hair follicle - a group of epidermal cells responsible for that hair's growth. The whole life of a hair depends on the condition of its follicle, which in turn is largely determined by the level of blood circulation. If blood supply is impaired for some reason, shed hairs aren't re-placed by new ones. The tip of our head has lower blood circu-lation compared to other parts of the scalp. In majority of the cases, hair first starts getting sparse in that area, which is an indication that poor blood supply is the main cause of balding.

Men's hair becomes progressively sparser as they advance in years because blood circulation in their scalps decreases. A forty-year-old male has much lower blood circulation compared to what it was in his twenties. The network of capillary vessels loses its ability to nourish the scalp. Almost all men who start balding make the same mistake - they avoid touching their scalp because they think it would cause additional hair shedding. When combing and brushing, they are careful not to pull their hair or rub the skin. However, rubbing and massaging are the best ways to improve blood circulation in any part of the body. It's good to massage the scalp, especially in those areas where hair starts getting thin. We should follow the example of our women in this regard - they adjust, pull, comb, brush, and re-arrange their hair countless times every day, trying to look their best. Such behavior is really helpful in promoting good blood supply to the scalp. On top of that, thanks to estrogens present in their bodies, females are much less likely to suffer from circulatory disorders.

There is no proof that any ingredients from shampoos, creams, or conditioners can be absorbed by hair follicles. One of our skin's functions is preventing foreign substances from entering our body. Only some fats can be absorbed by the top layers of our skin. Even though the hair shaft is porous and can absorb chemical formulas (dyes, highlights, etc.), it doesn't mean that the shaft can transfer anything to the follicle - it is not possible to nourish the follicle from the outside. Nobody has so far found a way to deliver vitamins or nutrients to the follicles and stimulate hair re-growth.

Balding men can hold on longer to the hair on the sides of their head and in the occiput area because these areas don't have as many circulation-influencing factors. Some of those factors are related to the muscle and fat tissues under the scalp. The contraction of muscles (e.g. due to stress) can cause capillary vessels to contract, reducing blood supply to the follicles. Some men become bald as a result of their stressful life, full of nervous strain, causing their scalp to stay tense most of the time. Their undernourished hair follicles aren't able to re-grow hair.

In addition to rich supply, good blood quality is also important for healthy hair growth, and that is related to proper nutrition. It's been noticed that men who eat a lot of meat tend to lose hair on the top of their head, while those indulging in sweets usually start balding in the forehead area. Clean, healthy blood guarantees overall good health, which becomes reflected in the condition of our hair. Here are some basic steps to achieve that goal:

1. Prevent polluting your body by unhealthy diet.
2. Maintain healthy cholesterol levels allowing good blood circulation.
3. Use body-cleansing therapies, alternate hot and cold showers, fresh-air activities, and breathing exercises.

All these measures promote the health of your circulatory system. If you need more detailed information about them, find it in my other book, "Can we live 150 years?" Here, I'm only going to say more about scalp massage, a method which can give you a 90% chance to reverse your hair loss.

Head massage

The hardest part in teaching this method is convincing a person about the necessity to massage and brush his balding scalp. You can talk to hairstylists or dermatologists to find out, that

a bald spot never grows bigger as a result of massaging.
The towel used for the massage should be small and soft.

Remedy #52

Dissolve 2 tablespoons of salt in 1qt (1L) of warm water,
soak a towel in the solution, wring it gently, and massage
affected parts of your scalp. Pay particular attention to areas where there is only partial hair loss. You decide for yourself the length of the massage - for example, when the skin
takes on a rosy color or when there is a stinging sensation.
It might take anywhere from half a minute to several minutes.

The goal is to gradually restore the network of capillary vessels in our scalp to good condition, which in turn would regenerate our hair follicles. Please do not expect immediate results - the problem took years to build up and the remedy is
going to take at least as long, but the effort can pay off if you
are patient. The first re-grown hairs are likely to show in 3-4
months. When the bald spot starts losing its smoothness, it is
the sign of follicles pushing new hair shafts up to the surface.
Visually, some types of hairs might be noticeable sooner, depending on their color or the shape of hair shafts. For example,
dark hair shows up sooner than fair one, even if they are re-
growing at the same rate.

You are going to shed some hairs during the massage. These are the ones that are ready to fall out anyway. In about three
month's time, their rejuvenated follicles will start pushing up
new hairs. Even a very intense massage cannot remove hairs
that are not meant to be shed. The process of thinning is stopped and reversed as soon as you start massage therapy. There
will be more new hairs growing than the old ones shed, until
the area returns to normal hair thickness. It usually takes one

to five years - about as long as the thinning has been allowed to go on. Please don't stop massaging until the full re-growth takes place.

Re-growing hair in cases of complete baldness is a separate question. It's theoretically possible, but I wouldn't like to make vain promises. Trying is not going to hurt you, but there is no guarantee as in the case of thinning hair.

People who reverse the process of hair thinning are advised to maintain the massaging habit for the rest of their lives. Even those who have never had any problems with their hair but expect them due to genetic factors, poor nutrition, or stressful lifestyle, can use scalp massage as a preventative measure. Such head start with the therapy will guarantee full and thick hair on your head.

Daily hair washing cannot cause any extra shedding. You wash your face even more frequently and it doesn't cause to lose your eyebrows or eyelashes. Some experts advise against daily hair washing and say it dries your hair up by removing natural oils secreted by skin glands. In my opinion, removing that fatty material together with dust stuck to it is actually a good idea. Daily washing combined with head massage helps regulate the functioning of skin glands, which also influences our hair's condition. In order to maintain soft, manageable hair and well-functioning skin glands, you can use an egg yolk in your wash and then follow it by 1-2 minutes of massage. Drinking alcohol in small amounts (25-50mL a day) also promotes healthy hair growth by expanding our capillary vessels. Don't forget about sex, it also helps provide richer blood supply to the hair follicles, just like all other activities relaxing our nervous system.

Here are a few additional methods that can help you accelerate the process of follicle rejuvenation.

Remedy #53

Ingredients: 3.5oz (100g) of nettle leaves (best harvested in May)

Preparation: Pour 0.5qt/500mL of boiling water on the leaves, let the brew stand for 30min, strain, and soak a towel in it.

Usage: Massage your scalp with the towel.

Remedy #54

Ingredients: Table salt

Usage: Rub on your scalp for 10-12 minutes, let it remain that way for 1 hour, then rinse off the salt and massage your scalp. Use this method once a week.

Remedy #55

Ingredients: 1 teaspoon of brandy, 1 teaspoon of corn oil, 1 teaspoon of kefir

Preparation: Blend the ingredients.

Usage: Rub the mixture on your scalp, cover it with a plastic bag, and put a toque on top of it for 15-20 minutes. Rinse your hair thoroughly and massage your scalp.

Remedy #56

Ingredients: 0.5L of grated red beets

Preparation: Put the beets into a 1L jar and fill the jar with boiled water. Cover the jar with a lid and let it ferment at room temperature for 5 days, then strain liquid out of it.

Usage: Rub the liquid on your scalp once a day, until it's used up. After 2 months, repeat the therapy.

Now that you know how to deal with hair loss, start massaging your scalp today. This way, like many of my patients, you may have a good reason to rejoice in front of the mirror four months from now.

Closing Advice

1. Love yourself the way you are.
2. Do not envy anybody.
3. If you do not like yourself, make changes in your life.
4. Anger, insults, and criticism of yourself and others are very harmful to your health.
5. If you make a decision, act on it.
6. Joyfully help the poor, ill, and elderly.
7. Never think about diseases, old age, or death.
8. Love is the best remedy against illness and aging.
9. Gluttony, greed, and inability to overcome your weaknesses are your enemies.
10. Worrying causes you to leave this world.
11. Fear and corruption are the worst sins.
12. The best day of your life is today.
13. The best town is where you feel fortunate.
14. The best occupation is the one you enjoy.
15. Losing hope is the worst mistake.
16. The greatest gift you can give or receive is love.
17. Health is your most valuable possession.

Appendix A

Diseases from A to Z

Alcoholism

Abuse of alcohol brings a lot of pain and suffering, affecting not only to the abuser but also to his family and friends. In dealing with stressful life situations, some people repeatedly turn to a strong drink in order to "unwind" their nervous tension. Unlike moderate alcohol consumption, such abuse damages our health and destroys relationships.

There is a very wise ancient saying:

> *There are three things that are very harmful when used excessively and very beneficial in moderate amounts - bread, salt, and wine.*

I wrote earlier about bread and salt. Let's take a look at wine.

Since our childhood, we hear much about the harmful effects of alcohol consumption - I would not be able to say anything new about that. I suggest we also consider some health benefits of moderate alcohol consumption.

Once I have seen an interesting cartoon. Animals in the Kalahari Desert gathered to have a meal together. Berries used for the meal were partially fermented. As an effect of eating the berries, the animals became very peaceful - predators and prey, lions and antelopes, tigers and elephants were all very happy and forgot about hatred and aggression. It turns out that mammals (including humans, the most developed ones) need small amounts of alcohol. It causes our brain to release "the hormone of happiness", relaxing the muscles, lowering our concentration and the tension of our nervous system. We receive all these benefits only if we use alcohol in small amounts, treating it like a medication. Hippocrates also believed that alcohol in moderate amounts is appropriate for both the healthy and the ill.

In the opinion of Louis Pasteur, wine has the full right to be considered the healthiest of all beverages if used with moderation. Ancient Greek philosophers often repeated to their followers: "The power of gods can hardly equal the usefulness of wine," and the old Eastern adage says: "Everybody can drink as long as they know the right time, place, amount, and can afford it."

This kind of reasoning can be found in the opinions of many respected thinkers. Our troubles begin when we forget about moderation. This applies to all aspects of life, not only to eating and drinking.

Determining what we mean by "moderate amount" is more complicated - it can have different meanings for different people. American researchers, based on many years of studies, suggest the following amounts as harmless: 1g of wine or 0.25g of liquor per 1kg of body weight a day. Different kinds of wine influence our health differently. For example, white wine cleanses the kidneys, slightly stimulates the nervous system, and improves digestion. Red wine improves the functioning of our liver, calms the nervous system, improves breathing processes, and lowers the risk of heart disease in people with high cholesterol level.

The information presented below can be useful for anybody - from abstainers to heavy drinkers. Studies conducted in different countries reached some common conclusions about the influence of drinking wine on different systems in our body:

1. It positively affects the nervous system and stimulates the endocrine glands.
2. It improves digestion (of animal protein in particular) by stimulating the secretion of gastric juices.
3. It helps maintain the proper pH level of the gastric juices.
4. By positively influencing the digestive system, it slightly relieves the stress on the entire body.
5. Liver cells stimulated by alcohol supply more bile to the duodenum.
6. Potassium salts present in wine and brandy have a diuretic effect on the kidneys.
7. Stimulated breathing centers improve the ventilation of the lungs.
8. It improves the cardiovascular system by causing the vessels to expand and contract, which has a massaging effect.
9. Alcohol flushes toxic products (e.g. phenol) out of the body.
10. The delicate aroma stimulates our smell centers.
11. Alcohol has disinfecting and antitoxic qualities.
12. It prevents the accumulation of fat on the walls of blood vessels, reducing the risk of cardiovascular disorders.

There have been many studies in recent years concerning the influence of alcohol on the heart muscle. Some researchers concluded that every beverage containing alcohol strengthens the heart. They particularly point out the high content of natural antioxidants in red wine. It was noticed that people who never consume any alcoholic beverages suffer much more frequently from heart disorders. English and Swiss scientists concluded that alcohol in moderate amounts reduces the risk of heart attacks by 40% and the disorders of blood vessels by 20%.

I would like to stress that wine drinking is particularly beneficial for the elderly and for people suffering from anemia or weak health in general.

There is a saying in Burgundy: "Wine is the milk for the elderly." It is advisable for people over fifty to prepare and consume the "longevity drink" once a week (best on Sunday with a group of good friends). It is especially helpful for women going through menopause.

"Longevity drink" preparation: In a pot, mix two bottles of sweet or semi-sweet wine with 0.5 liter of water. Boil it for 10 minutes using low heat; add a pinch of clove buds, cinnamon, and cardamom, and 10 slices of peeled lemon and then boil for another 5 minutes. Finally add one tablespoon of brandy, turn off the heat, cover the pot with a lid, and let it stand for 20 minutes. Strain the mixture and drink while it is still warm (this recipe is for 10 servings - divide the amounts by 10 if you want to prepare just one serving).

Lack of moderation can lead to dependency, which should be treated as a disease. Alcoholics don't usually want to admit that, neither are they willing to undergo treatment. Their body becomes used to the poison and demands regular doses of it. Body cleansing routines help break that vicious cycle. When alcoholics have clean blood circulating in their system, they are able to think clearly about the serious consequences of continued dependency and the harm they bring on themselves and their close ones. Breaking out of the denial mode is a major step, but lack of strong will often prevents sustained effort needed for full recovery. Here, family and friends have to step and provide understanding together with compassionate support.

Those who are ready to deal with the addiction can try the following remedy.

Remedy #57
Break up 4 laurel leaves and put them into a 0.5qt (0.5L) bottle of vodka. Let it stand in a dark place for 14 days. When you try to drink it, you'll experience intense vomiting, which should result in disgust to alcohol.

If an alcoholic cannot accept the seriousness of the situation and the necessity for treatment on the conscious level, somebody close can try another method, which contains elements of hypnosis. This can work even in cases where the addict isn't willing to make any effort towards recovery. Directions received in the sleep state work on the subconscious level. I have used the method in my practice and consider it one of the most effective in treating alcoholism. The same general idea can be used to stop certain other problems, e.g. nail biting, bed wetting, or sleepwalking in the case of children. We have to be patient in our effort, even if we need to try several times before we see results.

Remedy #58

There are two stages in this therapy.

Stage 1

Before your "subject" goes to bed (e.g. during supper), say to him the following words, "I'll come and talk to you about something very important when you are asleep." Say it in a normal tone, without emphasis.

Stage 2

When the "subject" is asleep, walk up quietly and start gently stroking his hair. Start talking to him, using his name, e.g. "Can you hear me, Matthew?" Even if there's no response, keep talking and stroking the "subject's" hair, as if you were sharing a problem with a friend. After about 5 minutes, touch the "subject's" temples using the thumb and the middle finger of your right hand. You should be able to feel the pulse in the temporal arteries. At this point, you can start entering your suggestion by repeatedly telling the "subject" what he needs to give up, for example, "Matthew, you're going to quit drinking tomorrow. When you get up in the morning, forget about that habit. It has never done you any good." Use your imagination in creating suggestions. The last phrase can be something like, "Have a good sound sleep and when you are well rested, wake up happy and forget about your addiction. If necessary, I'll come back and talk to you about it again, until you are able to take this step." Quietly leave the bedroom.

Note: If the "subject" wakes up when you touch his hair, just keep stroking his hair and talking quietly. When you hear deep regular breathing again, return to entering your suggestion. I only present here a general idea of how the therapy can be done. Your own intuition and knowledge of your "subject's" personality will allow you to create the best method for your specific needs.

Anemia

Note: Please carefully read information about the properties of fruit and vegetable juices (see "Can We Live 150 Years?" p. 83-85).

Remedy #59
Ingredients: Beet juice
Usage: Drink half a cup 6 times a day for 3-4 weeks.

Remedy #60
Ingredients: 3 large beets
Preparation: Grate the beets, put in a 0.5L jar and pour 5.3oz (150g) of vodka on them. Let it stand exposed to sunlight or in a warm place for 14 days and then filter the liquid out.
Usage: Drink 1oz (30g) of the liquid before meals. If your blood composition doesn't improve, repeat the therapy.

Remedy #61
Ingredients: Aloe Vera juice 5.3oz (150g), honey 250g, red wine 350mL
Preparation: Blend the ingredients.
Usage: Drink 1oz (30g) of the mixture 3 times a day, 20 minutes before meals.

Remedy #62
Ingredients: Herbal tea brewed from wild strawberry leaves
Usage: Drink 3-4 glasses daily.

Remedy #63
Ingredients: Herbal tea brewed from nettle leaves (best if

harvested in May)
Usage: Drink 3-4 glasses daily.

Remedy #64

Eggshell therapy - see page 31

Remedy #65

Ingredients: Freshly squeezed carrot, beet, and black radish juices
Preparation: Blend in equal amounts.
Usage: Take 2 tablespoons a day for 3 months.

Arrhythmia

Remedy #66

Ingredients: Grated lemons 500g, honey 500g, 20 ground
Preparation: Blend the ingredients.
Usage: Take 1 tablespoon before breakfast and supper.

Arteriosclerosis

> Drink half a cup of juice squeezed from raw potatoes on an empty stomach in the morning for 14 days.
> Take a lemon therapy.
> Cleanse your liver.
> Eat 1 grapefruit on an empty stomach in the morning and 1 in the evening two hours after your last meal.
> Drink 2-3 cups of green tea every day.
> Cleanse your lymphatic system.
> Cleanse your blood.
> Use Nishi exercise set. (p. 117-119)
> Take alternate hot and cold showers in the morning and the afternoon.

> Drink 1/3 cup of pumpkin juice, a cup of watermelon juice, or 1/3 cup of beet juice 3 times a day, 15 minutes before meals.

Remedy #67
Ingredients: 9oz (250g) of horseradish; 3qt (3L) water
Preparation: Wash and grate about 9oz (250g) of horseradish. Pour 3qt (3L) of boiling water on it, boil for another 20 minutes, and then strain.
Usage: Drink half a cup 3 times a day

Remedy #68
Ingredients: Grapefruit; olive oil.
Preparation: Mix juice from half a grapefruit and mix it with 1 tablespoon of olive oil.
Usage: Take everyday for one month and make one-month interval before repeating. Use this therapy once a year

Remedy #69
Preparation: Grind and mix walnuts, raisins, honey, and figs - 3.5oz (100g) each.
Usage: Take 1 tablespoon or as a spread twice a day.

Remedy #70
Ingredients: Juice from 2 large heads of garlic and 8.8oz (250g) of vodka
Preparation: Pour vodka on top of garlic juice in a half-liter jar and let it stand in a dark place for 12 days.
Usage: Take 20 drops 3 times a day (30 minutes before meals) for 3 weeks. Take a month interval; repeat for another 3 weeks, and so on until the supply is finished.

Remedy # 71

Ingredients: 1 tablespoon of corn flour
Preparation: Put in a cup, fill the cup with boiling water, and let it stand for 10 hours (overnight).
Usage: Drink on the empty stomach (clear brew only) in the morning.

Remedy #72

Ingredients: 1 cup of carrot juice, 1 cup of grated horseradish, 1 cup of honey, juice from 1 lemon
Preparation: Mix the ingredients, pour in a bottle, and store refrigerated.
Usage: Take 1 teaspoon 3 times a day.

Arthritis

Remedy #20 page 70
Remedy #9 page 67
Remedy #18 page 69
Remedy #19 page 70

Ascaris (intestinal parasites)

Remedy #73

Ingredients: 1 onion
Preparation: Chop the onion finely, pour a cup of boiling water on it, let it stand for 12 hours, and strain juice out of it.
Usage: Drink 1 cup daily for 5-7 days.

Remedy #74

Eat 200g of pumpkin seeds on an empty stomach.

Remedy #75
Ingredients: 1 cup of milk, 10 peeled cloves of garlic
Preparation: Put garlic in a pot, pour milk on it, slowly heat to the point of boiling, let it stand long enough to cool off, and strain it.
Usage: Drink the milk. Half an hour later use an herbal laxative. Three hours after that, perform an enema (intestinal irrigation) using 200mL of warm water.

Remedy #76
Drink up to 1 qt (1 L) of freshly squeezed carrot juice every day.

Remedy #77
Ingredients: Onion, vodka
Preparation: Take a 200mL bottle, fill it in half with finely chopped onion, top it up with vodka, let it stand in a dark warm place for 12-14 days, and strain liquid out of it.
Usage: Take 1 tablespoon of the liquid 3 times a day before meals.

Remedy #78
Another effective method which can also be safely used by children is drinking a cup of juice squeezed out of pumpkin pulp every morning on an empty stomach.

<u>Bloating</u>

In order to prevent gases from forming, you need first to perform large intestine cleansing (see p. 141). Paying attention to proper combinations of food types in your meals is also very important (see Table 2, p. 52) because incompletely digested sugars and starch moving from the small intestine to the large intestine cause fermentation and gas formation. Those suffering from cardiovascular problems should especially avoid bloating, because inflated intestines can lead to a heart attack. There are several ways to deal with bloating.

1. Chamomile enema (in case of sudden bloating with abdominal pains): Brew 200mL of chamomile tea using 1 teaspoon or 1 teabag of chamomile. Add it to 1.5qt (1.5L) of boiled water cooled down to body temperature and use this solution to perform intestinal irrigation (see p. 141). After that, lie on your back for 30-40 minutes with a thermal pad covering your stomach and liver area.

2. Juice squeezed from raw potatoes is a wonderful remedy against bloating and other digestive tract problems. Drink 100mL on the empty stomach in the morning every day for 2 weeks, take a 2-week interval, and then continue for another 2 weeks. If this doesn't take care of the problem, drink it for another 10 days (following another 2-week interval).

3. Brew 400mL of eucalyptus tea by pouring boiling water on a handful of eucalyptus leaves, and drink it warm on the empty stomach.

Burns

➤ Put finely grated carrot on the affected area.

➤ Mix an egg yolk with a teaspoon of butter (it should resemble mayonnaise), put on a soft pad and apply on the affected area. It will relieve pain and prevent scars.

➤ Rinse the affected area under cold water and generously apply baking soda. In case of burns in the throat, rinse it with 1 tablespoon of oil and swallow the oil.

Bone, joint, and muscle pains

See page 67-71

Bronchial asthma

For any remedy to be effective, the cervical and thoracic vertebrae have to be correctly aligned. To stop a sudden asthma
attack, you can give the affected person small ice cubes to swallow, a coffee bean to chew on, or barley-based coffee substitute to drink. Lying face up on a hard floor, while having the
shoulders massaged, also helps stop an attack. Hypnotherapy
has proved itself very effective in dealing with asthma. You
can also try the following remedies.

Remedy # 79
Ingredients: 1 cup of black radish juice
Preparation: Boil the juice and then let it cool off.
Usage: Drink 1 cup 15 minutes before meals.

Remedy # 80
Ingredients: Butter 3.5oz (100g), 5-8 squeezed-out garlic
cloves, a pinch of salt
Preparation: Mix the ingredients
Usage: Spread on a slice of bread and eat.

Remedy #81 (to treat early stages of asthma in children)
Ingredients: 5 crushed aspirin pills, 1 tablespoon of lard
Preparation: Mix the ingredients
Usage: Spread on a piece of fabric and put on the child's
chest for 10 days in a row.

Remedy #82
   Ingredients: 40 average-size onions, 1 qt (1 L) of olive oil
   Preparation: Pour boiling water on the onions and let them
   stand long enough to become tender, then cook them in oil
   till softness, and crush into a pulp.
   Usage: Take 1 tablespoon in the morning on the empty stomach and 1 tablespoon in the evening. Store refrigerated. You
   may warm up before use.

Bronchitis

If you experience coughing due to bronchitis, avoid coffee and
tea, because they irritate respiratory passages. You can drink
herbal teas or milk with some honey and a pinch of baking
soda. Use pasteurized honey because raw honey can increase
your coughing.

For acute bronchitis, use one of the following remedies:

Remedy # 83
   Ingredients: 1 cup of freshly squeezed carrot juice, 2 table-
   spoons of honey
   Preparation: Blend the ingredients.
   Usage: Take 2 tablespoons 5-6 times a day.

Remedy #84
   Ingredients: 1 cup of freshly squeezed cabbage juice, 2
   tablespoons of honey
   Preparation: Blend the ingredients.
   Usage: Take 1 tablespoon 4 times a day.

Remedy #85
   Ingredients: 1 tablespoon of dried lime tree flowers, 1 table-

spoon of honey
Preparation: Pour 1 cup of boiling water on the flowers, add honey, let it stand for 1 hour, then strain it.
Usage: Drink 1 cup 3-4 times a day.

For chronic bronchitis, try these cough-inducing remedies:

Remedy #86
Ingredients: Bran 400g
Preparation: Boil 1.5L of water, add bran, cook on low heat for 5 minutes, then let it cool off and strain it.
Usage: Drink throughout the day. You can add some sugar to improve taste. It's a good idea not to drink any other fluids.

Remedy #87
Ingredients: 1 tablespoon of raspberry jam, 1 tablespoon of honey, 1 tablespoon of vodka or brandy, juice from half a lemon
Preparation: Mix in a cup and fill with boiling water.
Usage: Drink in small sips before going to bed.

Remedy #88
Ingredients: Juice from one lemon, 3.5oz (100g) of honey
Preparation: Blend the ingredients.
Usage: Take 1 tablespoon 3 times a day.

Remedy #89
Ingredients: Dried lime tree flowers 3.5oz (100g), dried raspberries 3.5oz (100g)
Preparation: Pour 1L of boiling water on the ingredients, let it stand for a while, and strain the brew.
Usage: Drink warm before going to bed, 7oz (200g) 1.8oz (50g) a day for 2-3 days.

Remedy #90
  Ingredients: Radish juice, horseradish juice, and honey - 1 cup each
  Preparation: Blend, boil, and let it stand for 3-4 hours.
  Usage: Take 3 times a day, 1 hour after each meal (adults - 2 tablespoons, children - 1 teaspoon).

Remedy #91
  Ingredients: Grated onion 1.8oz (50g), vinegar 0.7oz (20g), honey 2oz (60g)
  Preparation: Pour vinegar on the onion, squeeze and filter liquid out of the mixture, and blend the liquid with honey.
  Usage: Take 1 tablespoon every half hour.

Remedy #92
  Ingredients: Grated onion 3.5oz (100g), sugar crystals 3.5oz (100g)
  Preparation: Shake sugar on the onion, let it stand for a while, and squeeze liquid out.
  Usage: Take 2 teaspoons 3 times a day.

Remedy #93
  Ingredients: Garlic, honey
  Preparation: Crush some garlic and mix with equal amount of honey.
  Usage: Take 1 teaspoon 3 times a day or 1 tablespoon before going to bed. Drink some warm water with it.

Remedy #94
  Ingredients: 1 bottle of beer, 1 tablespoon of honey
  Preparation: Pour the beer in a pot, add honey, and boil for 5 minutes.
  Usage: Drink warm during coughing attacks.

Remedy #95

Ingredients: A few radishes, sugar crystals
Preparation: Wash the radishes, carve holes in them, and fill the holes with sugar. After at least 40 minutes squeeze juice out.
Usage: Take 1 teaspoon 3 times a day.

Constipation

There are many potential causes of constipation and it's up to you to try and select the most effective remedy from the list below. Sporadic occurrence of constipation can be caused simply by your stomach's contents becoming stagnant, and then it's enough to restrain from eating any food and to drink only half a glass of warm boiled water every 1-1.5 hour throughout the day until the problem disappears. Chronic constipation, without bowel movement for 36 or more hours at a time, is much more dangerous and can potentially cause a range of health problems, from headaches to strokes. The most effective strategy involves large intestine irrigation (enema) and re-establishing of healthy intestinal flora. Some other methods that can be helpful are listed below.

> ➢ Eat 2 apples with the peel on the empty stomach in the morning.
> ➢ Eat 2 oranges before bedtime. Peel of only the outer layer (1mm), leaving the fruit's white under-skin.
> ➢ Pour 1.5 cup of boiling water on 2 teaspoons of bran, cover with a lid, let it stand overnight, and eat the bran in the morning. Continue for 10-14 days.
> ➢ Put 5-6 dried plums in 1 cup of kefir and let it stand for 8-10 hours. Drink the kefir and eat the plums before bedtime every day for 30 days.

> Drink 1 glass of cold water on the empty stomach in the morning for 7 days.
> Pour 1 cup of boiling water on 1 teaspoon of flaxseed. Drink together with the seeds before bedtime (14 days at the most, don't use flaxseed if you suffer from chronic liver problems).
> Take 1 tablespoon of oil on the empty stomach in the morning and before bedtime.
> Drink 1 cup of carrot juice on the empty stomach in the morning and before bedtime.
> Drink 1 cup of raw potato juice on the empty stomach in the morning and before bedtime.
> Alternately deflate and inflate your abdomen 20-40 times while still lying in bed in the morning.
> Consume more products that promote healthy intestine function: fruits and vegetables in all forms, salty and sour foods (e.g. sauerkraut, pickled cucumbers), honey, rye bread, buckwheat, and white wine.
> Limit your consumption of coffee, tea, hot soups, cocoa, white bread, sweet biscuits and other white flour products, fatty meat, smoked products, and sweet beverages.

Diabetes Pages 144-145

Eczema

After shower, rub a mixture of equal amounts of sunflower oil and apple cider vinegar on the affected areas.

Eye disorders

Grate an apple or potato, mix it with an egg white, and put on the eyes. Rinse off with warm boiled water.

Excessive night sweating

Rub apple cider vinegar on your skin before going to bed.

Flu

The best antibiotics given us by nature are found in onion, garlic, lemon, and grapefruit. Remedies involving any of these products or turnips, parsley, and raspberry leaves can be used in dealing with flu. The fundamental strategy is drinking a lot of freshly squeezed juices and taking homemade formulas based on garlic and onion. Eat less, drink and exercise more, and most important, make sure to sweat as much as possible out of your body. Cleanse your large intestine by irrigation (enema) as soon as you become ill. You can use regular enema only (1-1.5qt/1-1.5L of water plus juice squeezed from one lemon) for seven days, or alternate it with garlic enema. Simply pour a cup of boiling water on 3-4 garlic cloves, then strain it and use the liquid for your enema.

Note: In order to prevent getting ill during the flu season, you can use the following formula every day between October and April. Grate two lemons (remove the seeds), peel and chop up two heads of garlic, mix everything well, and pour 1.5qt (1.5L) of boiled water on it. Let it stand for three days in a dark place at room temperature, then strain liquid out and store it in the refrigerator. Take one tablespoon on the empty stomach in the morning and one before bedtime (one teaspoon in the case of children). If you follow this diligently, the probability of catching a flu will be very slim.

It's also a good idea to perform nose irrigation. Dissolve 1 teaspoon of salt and 1 teaspoon of baking soda in 1 cup of warm water, and then add 5 drops of iodine. Use the solution to alternately irrigate both nostrils.

You can use the following garlic formula for prevention during flu outbreaks:

Remedy #96
Ingredients: 2 or 3 garlic cloves, 1-1.7 fl oz (30-50mL) of boiling water.
Preparation: Chop the garlic finely, pour boiling water over it, and let it stand 1-2 hours, and strain (store for up to 2 days, keep refrigerated).
Usage: Use as nose drops 1 or 2 times a day - 2 or 3 drops into each nostril.

➢ To avoid infecting your family, you can hang a small cotton bag with finely chopped garlic on your neck (2 or 3 cloves). To protect small children from the outbreak, put such cotton bag or a small plate with chopped garlic next to their beds.

➢ Another way of flu prevention is chewing a eucalyptus leaf every morning and keeping a piece of such leaf in your mouth (between the gum and the cheek) during contacts with flu-infected people. You can also rinse your throat every evening with freshly squeezed raw beet juice blended with a teaspoon of 3% vinegar.

Use the following advice if you cannot prevent the infection and become ill.

➢ Drink hot tea with lemon (or raspberry jam) or warm milk with honey (1 tablespoon per cup) as often as possible.

➢ Heat up some chamomile essence and breathe the vapors in.

➢ Put cotton swabs dipped in fresh onion juice into your nostrils for seven minutes 3-4 times a day.

➤ Squeeze an onion into a little bowl and sniff the juice for 2-3 minutes 3 times a day.

➤ Grate finely a head of garlic and mix with an equal amount of honey (lime honey is best). Take 1 tablespoon before bedtime and drink some warm water.

➤ Grate an onion, pour 0.5 quart (0.5L) of boiling milk over it and store in a warm place. Drink hot - half of it before bedtime and half in the morning.

➤ Pour 1 cup of boiling water over 2 tablespoons of dried (or 3.5oz/100g of fresh) raspberries. Let it stand for 10-15 minutes, add 1 tablespoon of honey, and mix well. Take warm before bedtime to stimulate sweating.

➤ Pour boiling water over a mixture (1:1) of dried lime flowers and raspberries (1 cup of water per 1 tablespoon of the mixture). Wrap the pot in a towel for 1 hour and then strain it. Drink 1 cup of the brew 3-4 times a day.

➤ Pour 0.5qt (0.5L) of boiling water over a pinch of a mixture (1:1) of dried lime flowers and blackcurrant leaves. Boil it for another 5 minutes, wrap the pot in a towel for half and hour, and then strain the brew. Drink 1 cup 3-4 times a day, warm like a tea.

Furuncles (boils)

Make a small loaf out of some flour, fresh milk, and fresh butter. Put it on the affected spot and leave there overnight. This should make the "core" of the furuncle come out.

Fungal infections

Remedy #97 (against fungal infections under fingernails or toenails)
  Ingredients: Ground coffee

Preparation: Pour boiling water over ground coffee (sufficient amount to make a strong brew), let it cool off, and pour into a basin together with the grinds.
Usage: Submerge affected areas in the brew several times a day.

Remedy #98 (to treat fungal infections around the toes)
Wash your feet thoroughly before going to bed, submerge them in wine vinegar, and wear socks soaked with wine vinegar overnight

Remedy #99 (to treat fungal infections around the toes)
Crush some mint leaves together with salt crystals into fine powder, and put it between your toes for 1 hour. Repeating this routine several times should completely eliminate the infection.

Headaches

There are some ways to stop headaches without taking any pharmaceuticals. Try the following methods.

> ➤ (For migraine headaches) Wear an amber necklace for a prolonged period of time.
> ➤ (For migraine headaches) Perform body-cleansing routines - at least for the large intestine, liver, and the lymphatic system.
> ➤ Put your feet (about 10cm deep) in a basin with hot water and drink a hot strong tea with 2 teaspoons of sugar or honey, or a hot mint leaf tea with 2 teaspoons of sugar.
> ➤ If your headache is caused by accumulation of gases in your abdomen, perform an enema (as recommended by Dr. Walker), then lie down and cover your liver area with

a thermal pad for 30-45 minutes.

➢ Plug your both ears with cotton swabs soaked in freshly squeezed beet or onion juice.

➢ Take an alternate hot and cold shower for 10-15 minutes. Start with a hot shower, moving gradually from your feet up to your head, then a cold shower in the same manner, and so on.

➢ Before going to bed, suck on a tablespoon of sugar and then drink a cup of warm boiled water.

➢ Massage your head, neck, and shoulders.

➢ If it feels like one of your nostrils has more difficulty letting the air through, plug the other nostril with a swab and cover it with your finger, breathing only through one nostril. This should take care of your headache in 15-20 minutes.

➢ Perform any set of spine-strengthening exercises, paying particular attention to the cervical section of your spine.

➢ Tap the top of your head alternately with your left and right palm (100 times each.

➢ Massage strongly your earlobes with your fingers, almost to the point of pinching.

Heartburn

Heartburn is caused by improperly combining food types. Different segments of our digestive tract secrete different digestive juices. As a result of incorrect food combination, incompletely digested food moves from our stomach to duodenum together with acidic gastric juice, which eventually leads to disorders of both the stomach and duodenum. Heartburn is a side effect of disturbed digestive functions. There are a few other important rules that help prevent heartburn.

> ➤ Chew your food slowly and thoroughly.
> ➤ Always eat in relaxed atmosphere, free of stress and anxiety.
> ➤ Try to eat only freshly prepared meals.
> ➤ Limit your intake of fatty and fried foods.
> ➤ Don't drink at your meals.

Several simple remedies can help you deal with heartburn.

> ➤ Lemon juice therapy is very effective (p. 40-42).
> ➤ Drink juice from one lemon blended with a powdered eggshell.
> ➤ For 14 days, eat only buckwheat for breakfast, on the empty stomach (make sure to chew it well).
> ➤ Dry up a tablespoon of buckwheat on the frying pan and grind it in your coffee grinder. Take a small amount (tip of a teaspoon) 3-4 times a day together with a few tablespoons of water.

Hemorrhoids

Hemorrhoids (dilated veins in the lower part of the large intestine) usually happen to people who habitually consume large amounts of bread, sweets, coffee, tea, and all kinds of sandwiches with bread and deli products.

Hemorrhoids are, among others, a sign of inefficient circulatory system, inflexible blood vessels and veins, and thickness of blood caused by deficiency in natural minerals found in vegetables and fruits. Contact of your anus with cold surfaces can also be a cause of hemorrhoids. Women often get hemorrhoids after child delivery and resulting dislocation of lumbar vertebrae.

Surgical removal of hemorrhoids benefits everybody involved except the patient. As a rule, hemorrhoids show up again after some time because the surgery does not remove their causes.

You can try a few therapies described below. Even though effective, they also are only a way to deal with the symptoms.

> Cut a stick (about as thick as your little finger) out of a raw potato and put in your rectum for the night. Use the therapy every other night for two weeks.
> Instead of using toilet paper after stools, wash your anus with alternately warm and cold water (five times each) and dry gently with a soft towel.
> Put 2 tablespoons of tobacco in a plastic bucket that is comfortable to sit on. Pour one quart (about 1L) of boiling water over it, put a lid on, and let it stand for 20 minutes. When the steam is not too hot anymore, take off the lid and sit on top of the bucket for 3-5 minutes.
> Drink the following juice blends 15 minutes before meals:
>   • 1.8oz (50g) carrot + 1.4oz (40g) celery + 0.7oz (20g) parsnips + 1.05oz (30g) spinach
>   • 3.2oz (90g) carrot + 2.1oz (60g) spinach
> Put an ice cube wrapped in cotton cloth into your rectum for 5-10 seconds. Use this therapy after stools (when you use a wash instead of toilet paper) for 1-2 months.

To get rid of hemorrhoids for good, switch to strictly fruit-and-vegetable diet for two weeks during summer months. Do not eat any meat, white flour products, or dairy products; do not drink coffee, cocoa, chocolate, or alcoholic beverages. You can eat small amounts of walnuts instead of bread and drink raspberry, currant, mint, or chamomile tea.

Finally, another important remark: suffering from hemorrhoids brings you a step closer to becoming ill with colon cancer.

High blood pressure

To reduce blood pressure, it is necessary to cleanse the circulatory system and the liver. Limit you intake of fats and flour-based products. Eat more foods rich in vitamin C and be more physically active.

Remedy #100
Ingredients: 1 cup of grated raw beets, 1 cup of honey
Preparation: Mix the ingredients.
Usage: Take 1 tablespoon 3 times a day 30 minutes before meals for 3 months.

Remedy #101
Ingredients: 2 cups of beet juice, 9oz (250g) of honey, juice from 1 lemon, 1 1 cup of blackcurrant juice, 1 cup of vodka
Preparation: Blend the ingredients.
Usage: Take 1 tablespoon 3 times a day 1 hour before meals.

Remedy #102
Ingredients: Juice from 6.6lb (3kg) of onions, 18oz (500g) of honey, seed partitions from 25 walnuts, 1 qt (1 L) of vodka
Preparation: Blend onion juice with honey, add walnut partitions, pour vodka over it, and let it stand in a dark place for 10 days.
Usage: Take 1 tablespoon 3 times a day.

Remedy #103
Ingredients: 0.5qt (0.5L) of vodka and 7oz (200g) of chopped garlic
Preparation: Pour vodka into a 0.75 quart (0.75L) dark glass bottle, add garlic, close tight, and let it stand in a dark place for 6-8 days (shake it from time to time). Strain the for-

mula, close tightly, and store refrigerated.
Usage: Take 1 tablespoon 3 times a day before meals.

Remedy #104

Ingredients: Seed partitions from 2.2lb (1kg) of walnuts, 1 qt (1 L) of vodka
Preparation: Put walnut partitions in a glass vessel, pour vodka on them, and let it stand until the color resembles strong dark tea
Usage: Take 1 tablespoon 3 times a day before meals.

Remedy #105

Ingredients: 20g of chopped garlic, 100g of sugar crystals
Preparation: Mix in a glass, fill with boiling water, stir well to completely dissolve sugar, and let it stand for 4-6 hours in a warm place. Store tightly closed in a dark place.
Usage: Take 1 tablespoon 3 times a day before meals.

Remedy #106

Take 1 teaspoon of honey mixed with cottage cheese 2-3 times a day.

Remedy #107

Drink a cup of tea with a tablespoon of honey daily before bedtime.

Remedy #108

Ingredients: 1 lemon without seeds, 7oz (200g) of cranberry, 7oz (200g) of wild rose fruit, 7oz (200g) of honey
Preparation: Put the lemon into boiling water for a while, dry it with a piece of cloth, and grate finely. Crush the cranberry and wild rose fruits. Put everything in a glass container, add honey, mix well, and let it stand for 24 hours.

Usage: Take 1 tablespoon 3 times a day 15 minutes before meals for 14-30 days.

Insomnia

Eating a lot of fruits and vegetables and drinking freshly squeezed juices is the best way to ensure good sleep. Another remedy you can try is taking some honey before going to bed. You can simply eat a tablespoon of honey, drink it dissolved in a cup of boiled water, drink one teaspoon dissolved in a cup of milk, or brew yourself half a cup of green tea with half a tablespoon of honey and 2 teaspoons of cream. Stuffing your pillow with eucalyptus leaves or hay can help you achieve restful sleep. Another simple thing to try is plugging your right nostril with a cotton swab and breathing only through the left nostril for at least 5 minutes. Two other remedies to deal with insomnia are given below.

Remedy #26 page 79

Remedy #109
  Ingredients: Dill seeds 50g, sweet red wine 1 qt (1 L)
  Preparation: Boil together for 1-2 minutes.
  Usage: Drink about 50mL before going to bed.

Kidney disorders

Remedy #110
  Ingredients: Pumpkin seeds 3.5oz (100g), flaxseed 3.5oz (100g)
  Preparation: Pour 1 qt (1L) of water on the pumpkin seeds, boil on low heat for 1 hour, and let it cool off. Pour 0.2qt (0.2L) of water on the flaxseed, boil for 20-30 minutes, and

make a compress out of it.

Usage: Drink the pumpkin seed brew, eat the pumpkin seeds, and use the flaxseed compress on your kidney area every day for a week.

Removing sand and stones from your kidneys

Remedy # 111

Ingredients: 1 tablespoon of chopped parsley greens, 1 tablespoon of chopped parsnips

Preparation: Pour 1 cup of boiling water on the ingredients and continue boiling on low heat for 1.5 hours. Strain the brew and divide into 3 equal parts.

Usage: Drink one part 3 times a day, 15 minutes before meals.

Remedy # 112

Ingredients: 1 tablespoon of flaxseed

Preparation: Pour 1 cup of water on the seeds, heat to the point of boiling, and strain.

Usage: Drink 1 cup a day for 7 days.

Remedy #113

Ingredients: 3 tablespoons of carrot seeds

Preparation: Put in a pot, pour 600mL of boiling water on it, wrap the pot in a towel, let it stand for 10 hours, and then strain.

Usage: Drink 1 cup 5-6 times a day until used up.

Remedy #114

Ingredients: Watermelon peel

Preparation: Chop up the peel, dry it in the oven, and grind into powder in a coffee grinder. Pour 50mL of boiling water on 1 teaspoon of the powder and let it cool off.

Usage: Drink 3-5 times a day until the condition is cured.

Remedy #115
Ingredients: 1 lemon (without seeds), 1.8oz (50g) of honey, 1.8oz (50g) of vegetable oil
Preparation: Put the lemon into boiling water for a moment, then dry it, grate, put in a glass container, add honey and oil, mix everything well, and cover with a lid.
Usage: Take 1 tablespoon 4-5 times a day.

Treating kidney stones, bladder stones, and urination problems

Remedy #116 (To prevent bladder and gallbladder stones)
Ingredients: Black radish, honey
Preparation: Grate the black radish and squeeze juice from it. Mix the juice with honey in equal amounts.
Usage: Drink half a cup once a day for a month.

Remedy #117
Ingredients: Juice squeezed from a horseradish (both root and leaves)
Usage: Take 1 teaspoon of freshly squeezed juice every morning and evening.

Remedy # 118
Ingredients: Carrot seeds
Preparation: Dry up the seeds on a frying pan and then grind them finely in a coffee grinder.
Usage: Take 1 teaspoon 3 times a day with 1 cup of water.

Remedy # 119
Ingredients: 2 dry parsnips

Preparation: Put the parsnips in a pot, pour 1 qt (1 L) of boiling water on them, and boil for another 3 minutes. Let the brew stand for 4 hours and then strain it.
Usage: Drink half a cup 3 times a day until the condition is cured.

Remedy #120
Ingredients: 1-11 tablespoons of chopped parsley greens
Preparation: Put the greens in a cup, fill with boiling water, cover with a lid, let it stand for 30 minutes, strain into a glass bottle, and close with a cork.
Usage: Drink 1 cup 3 times a day until the condition is cured.

Remedy #121
Ingredients: 3.5oz (100g) of unripe green walnuts (harvested before Jul 7) and 3.5oz (100g) of sugar crystals or honey
Preparation: Chop the walnuts finely, put them in a jar, add sugar or honey, close the jar tightly, and keep in the refrigerator for 1 month.
Usage: Take 1 teaspoon 3 times a day before meals. Store refrigerated.

Remedy #122
Ingredients: 3 lemons (with peel but without seeds), 5.3oz (150g) of peeled garlic, 0.5 quart (0.5L) of cool boiled water
Preparation: Grind lemon together with garlic, put in a 1 quart (1L) jar, fill the jar with water, let it stand 24 hours, strain it, close the jar tightly, and store in a dark place.
Usage: Drink 1.7 fl oz (50 mL) every morning.

Remedy #123
Ingredients: 3 cups of water, 4 lemons (without seeds), 1

cup of honey, and juice from 1 lemon

Preparation: Pour the water into a pot and add finely chopped lemons. Boil until there is only about 1 cup of brew left, let it cool off, strain it, pour in a glass container, add honey and lemon juice, mix well, and cover with a lid.

Usage: Take 1 tablespoon every day before bedtime until finished. Store refrigerated.

In case of kidney colic, put an electric heating pad on your kidney area or take a
hot bath.

Caution: Acute inflammations of other abdominal organs may cause similar
pains. If you are not sure that the pain is caused by kidney colic, do not follow
the advice given above and contact a physician.

How to prevent the formation of kidney stones?

➢ Pour 1 cup of boiling water on the peel from 1 apple, let it seep, and then drink it (twice a day).

➢ Drink 1oz (30g) of black radish juice on the empty stomach in the morning.

➢ Drink juice from 1 lemon blended with 1 tablespoon of olive oil on the empty stomach in the morning for 6 months.

Lack of appetite (children)

Remedy # 124

Ingredients: 4 teaspoons of raspberries

Preparation: Put in a thermos, fill with water, and let it stand for 2 hours.

Usage: Drink warm, half a cup 4 times a day.

Remedy #125
Ingredients: Celery juice
Usage: Take 2 teaspoons 3 times a day, 30 minutes before each meal.

Liver disorders

Remedy #126 (in case of liver pains)
Ingredients: 1 cup of olive oil, 1 cup of grapefruit juice
Preparation: Blend the juices.
Usage: Perform an enema in the evening, at least 2 hours after supper, and then drink the juice blend. Lie on your right side and put a thermal pad against your liver area. Repeat this routine every other day for a total of 3-5 times.

In order to relieve pain caused by an inflammation in your liver or gallbladder, try one of the following remedies.

Remedy #127
Ingredients: Cabbage juice
Usage: Drink 1 cup 3-4 times a day for 40 days.

Remedy #128
Ingredients: 2.2lb (1kg) of chopped onion, 2 cups of sugar
Preparation: Mix the ingredients, put the mixture in the oven, heat slowly until it produces yellow syrup, strain it out, and pour into a dark glass jar or bottle.
Usage: Take 1 tablespoon on the empty stomach, every morning for 3 months.

Remedy # 129
   Ingredients: Pumpkin juice
   Usage: Drink 1 cup twice a day before meals, for 30 days.

Remedy #130 (Stimulating the secretion of bile in cases
            of liver disorders)
   Ingredients: 3.5oz (100g) of wild rose fruits, some sugar
   Preparation: Put the wild rose fruit in a one-liter thermos,
   fill the thermos with boiling water, close it, and let it stand
   overnight.
   Usage: Drink the entire brew over 1 day adding some sugar
   for better taste.

Remedy #131 (Treating gallstones)
   Ingredients: A handful of dried birch leaves
   Preparation: Break up the leaves, pour 1 cup of boiling
   water over them, let the brew stand for 20 minutes (stir with
   a wooden spoon from time to time), and strain it.
   Usage: Take 1 cup of the brew before meals in the morning
   and the evening.

Remedy #132 (Treating gallstones)
   Ingredients: White cabbage
   Preparation: Chop the cabbage finely and squeeze juice
   out of it.
   Usage: Drink 1 cup at a time.

Remedy #133 (Treating gallstones)
   Ingredients: A black radish
   Preparation: Grate the radish and squeeze juice from it.
   Usage: Take 2-3 tablespoons of fresh juice every day.

Remedy #134 (Treating liver colic, liver stones)
   Ingredients: 10 dried figs, 1 cup of boiling water, 0.5 cup of hot milk, and 1 teaspoon of sugar
   Preparation: Chop the figs finely, put them in an enamel pot, pour boiling water over them, bring to the point of boiling, add milk and sugar, and let it cool off.
   Usage: Drink the liquid in small sips while still warm and eat the figs.

Low blood pressure

People with a tendency to low blood pressure should be physically active - walk and
run as much as possible.

➢ Pour 1 cup of boiling water on 1 teaspoon of black tea, cover it with a lid, and let seep for 5-7 minutes. Add 2 tablespoons of cream, a pinch of salt, and 1 teaspoon of sugar. Stir the brew and let it cool off. Drink for 7 days in the morning and the evening (10 minutes before meals), then take a 7-day interval. Repeat the cycle until your blood pressure goes back to normal.
➢ Regular use of sauna once a week for a year normalizes blood pressure.
➢ Alternate hot and cold showers wonderfully regulate the tone of blood vessels.
➢ Vibration massage helps increase blood pressure: Stand straight on your toes, your arms along your body, and then forcefully drop your body weight on your heels. Repeat 20 times in the morning and the evening. An alternate rhythmic stumping of your heels against the floor increases your blood pressure.
➢ Stomp your heels alternately against the floor (20-30 times

for each foot) in the morning and the evening. Continue the exercise daily until your blood pressure normalizes.

➤ "Goldfish" and "Cockroach" exercises from Nishi exercise set (p. 117-118) help regenerate your circulatory system. They not only correct low blood pressure problem but also improve your general health.

➤ If your blood pressure decreases during weather changes, drink at least 1 cup of carrot juice (four parts) mixed with beet juice (one part).

➤ Preventative lemon juice therapy (p. 40-41) can be used to increase low blood pressure.

Menopause

To delay menopause, use the following therapy starting at the age of forty:

Remedy #135

Ingredients: 7oz (200g) of white wine and 10-12 cloves of garlic.

Preparation: Slowly heat up wine to the point of boiling, add garlic and boil for another 30 seconds, let it cool off and pour in a dark glass bottle. Store in a dark place at room temperature.

Usage: Take 1 tablespoon 3 times a day 20 minutes before meals for 3 days in a row (day 1, 2, 3; 11, 12, 13; 21, 22, 23 of each month). The therapy also brings back the childbearing ability, improves skin complexion, and brings the sense of wellbeing.

Formula used to stop bleeding and eliminate unpleasant symptoms of menopause

Remedy #136

Ingredients: Peel from ten oranges, 2 quarts (2L) of boiling water, some sugar or honey

Preparation: Put orange peels in boiling water, cover the pot with a lid, and boil slowly until there is only about 0.7 quart (0.7L) of fluid left. Strain the brew twice and add sugar or honey for better taste. Pour the formula in a bottle and store refrigerated.

Usage: Take 1 tablespoon 3-4 times a day

Nipple inflammation

➢ Squeeze 2 white cabbage leaves enough to produce some juice, and put the leaves against your breasts for 1 to 3 hours.

➢ Mix 1 cup of flour with 1 tablespoon of honey, form the dough into a loaf, and cover the affected are with it for 40 to 60 minutes.

Obesity

Weight reducing diets:

➢ For 10 days, eat only different kinds of cereals (with some green leafy vegetables added). Cook your cereals in water with no salt added. You can eat up to 7 kinds of cereals a day without limiting the amounts. Limit your intake of fluids as much as possible. This allows you to lose 11-14.4lb (5-7kg) of excess weight.

➢ Maintain your usual diet, but chew each bite 100 times before it leaves your mouth. Drink only at least 15 minutes before and 2 hours after your meals. If you apply this strictly for a month, you can reduce your weight by

11-22lb (5-10kg).

➤ In the first week, eat only 2 oranges and 3 hard-boiled eggs (boil for about 12 minutes) 3 times a day. Enrich this diet in large amounts of raw fruits and vegetables in the second week.

➤ Drink 3 cup of freshly squeezed cabbage juice every morning and evening.

Swelling

In cases of swelling, it's a good idea to eat a lot of fruits and vegetables with diuretic (urination-inducing) properties, such as celery, parsley, asparagus, onion, garlic, watermelon, pumpkin, wild strawberries, and currants. Drinking 1 cup of pumpkin juice a day is also helpful.

Remedy #137
Ingredients: 2 average size onions, 1 tablespoon of sugar
Preparation: Cut the onions into thin slices, sprinkle with sugar, and leave overnight to produce juice, and squeeze the entire juice out.
Usage: Take 2 tablespoons a day.

Remedy # 138
Ingredients: 4 teaspoons of parsley seeds
Preparation: Pour 1 cup of boiling water on the seeds and let the brew stand for 8-10 hours.
Usage: Take 1 teaspoon 3-4 times a day 30 minutes before meals.

Remedy #139 (Swollen legs or abdomen)
Ingredients: Turnip peel
Preparation: Chop the peel finely and pour boiling water

on it (3 cups of water for 1 cup of peel). Cover the pot tightly, keep in low heat (without boiling) in the oven for 4 hours, and then strain it.
Usage: Drink 1 cup of the liquid daily.

Staphylococcus Aureus infection Remedy #40 page 134

Sore throat

Remedy #140
Ingredients: 1 lemon cut into small pieces
Usage: Suck on each lemon piece for 10 minutes, then swallow it (This is especially effective in the early stage.)

Remedy #141
Ingredients: White cabbage leaves
Usage: Put some leaves on your throat and wrap a woolen scarf around it. Replace with fresh leaves every 2 hours.

Remedy #142
Hold the right palm against your throat and the left against the temple of your head for 15-20 minutes. Repeat this daily for 3-5 days.

Remedy #143
Ingredients: Half a teaspoon of salt, half a teaspoon of baking soda, four drops of iodine
Preparation: Dissolve in a cup of boiled water.
Usage: Rinse your throat several times a day.

Remedy #144
Ingredients: 1 cup of beet juice, 1 tablespoon of apple cider vinegar or wine vinegar

Preparation: Blend the ingredients.
Usage: Rinse your throat 8-10 times a day.

Remedy #145
Ingredients: 3 teaspoons of broken up onion peels
Preparation: Put in a pot with 0.5L of water, boil, and then let it cool off.
Usage: Rinse your throat 5-6 times a day.

Remedy #146
Ingredients: 1 teaspoon of honey
Preparation: Dissolve in a cup of water.
Usage: Rinse your throat 8-10 times a day.

Remedy #147
Ingredients: Juice from 2 onions
Usage: Take 1 teaspoon 4 times a day.

Remedy #148
Ingredients: 1 apple, 1 onion
Preparation: Grate and blend.
Usage: Take 2 teaspoons 3 times a day.

Remedy #149
Ingredients: 1 red beet, 1 tablespoon of vinegar
Preparation: Grate the beet, add vinegar, let it stand for a few hours, and squeeze the liquid out into a glass vessel.
Usage: Use 1-2 tablespoons to rinse your throat, swallow afterwards.

Remedy #150
Ingredients: Milk 5.3oz (150g), 4-5 dried figs
Preparation: Pour the milk in a pot, add dried figs, and boil

for 5-7 minutes.
Usage: Drink in small sips (and eat the figs) before going to bed. Repeat for several days.

Remedy #151
Ingredients: 1 pear
Preparation: Wash, peel, and squeeze out juice.
Usage: Drink in small sips, holding in your mouth for a while before swallowing.

Thyroid gland disorders

➤ Wear an amber necklace.
➤ Soak pieces of oak tree bark in water and use the solution to make compresses on your throat. Apply this remedy for a prolonged period of time.
➤ Cover 2.2lb (1kg) of aronia berries (black chokeberries, Aronia melanokarpa) with 2.2lb (1kg) of sugar and let it stand in the refrigerator until it produces juice. Take 1 or 2 teaspoons 3 times a day.
➤ Grate one half of a lemon together with the peel, mix with 1 or 2 teaspoons of sugar, and eat the mixture (preferably 2 hours after a meal).
➤ Drinking 1 cup of lemon juice twice a day brings good results (see lemon juice therapy p. 40-42).

Appendix B

Healthy Recipes

Spring salads

Dandelion salad
Soak 3 handfuls of dandelion leaves in cool salty water to eliminate the bitter taste. Chop them up and mix with 10 ground walnuts. Add 1 tablespoon of sunflower oil or honey.

Radish and walnuts
Chop up or grate 15 radishes 3.5oz (100g), mix with 8 ground walnuts
(1.4oz/40g), add 1 teaspoon of vegetable oil and put some chopped chive on top.

French salad
Pour half a tablespoon of apple cider vinegar or wine vinegar over 3.5oz/100g of lettuce, add 1 tablespoon of vegetable oil and 1 teaspoon of chopped onion; mix everything well.

Young beet salad

Grate five or six young beets, add 2 tablespoons of cream, and season with a pinch of ground cumin.

Chive with peanuts

Chop up 1.8oz (50g) of chive and mix with 1.8oz (50g) of ground peanuts.

Radish with nuts, parsley, and mint

Grate 15 radishes, add a chopped parsley, some mint and dill, 0.5 of cumin, and 6 tablespoons 1.8oz (50g) of ground nuts.

Mix everything well. You can add some lettuce leaves as decoration.

Spinach salad

Chop up a handful of young spinach; add 1 tablespoon of chopped sorrel and 1 tablespoon of chopped chive; mix everything well. Add 3 tablespoons of ground peanuts and 1 tablespoon of bilberry.

Spinach and eggs

Whip up an egg yolk, gradually adding butter (1.5 tablespoon), then add 1 tablespoon of lemon juice. It should form a thick pulp when mixed. Add crushed garlic clove and 2 handfuls of chopped spinach. Mix again and put on a lettuce leaf.

Salad from beet leaves

Chop up young beet leaves (2 handfuls or about 2.1oz/60g). Prepare the sauce: Mix 1 egg yolk with 1 tablespoon of lemon juice, 0.5 teaspoon of mustard, 1 tablespoon of vegetable oil, and 1 teaspoon of chopped chive.

Summer and fall salads

Cucumbers and tomatoes

Mix chunks of cucumber with tomato slices; put 4 tablespoons of ground nuts on top.

Fresh cabbage salad

Mix 3.5oz (100g) of chopped cabbage with four tablespoons of grapefruit juice, 1 tablespoon of honey, and 0.5 teaspoon of cumin.

Peas and tomatoes

Mix 1.8oz (50g) of fresh peas with 4.2oz (120g) of crushed raw tomatoes and 2 tablespoons of sunflower oil. Put chopped parsley greens and chives on top.

Peas and carrots

Grate a carrot and mix it with 1.8oz (50g) of peas, 1 tablespoon of vegetable oil, 1 tablespoon of raspberry or currant juice, and chopped-up 0.5 of an onion.

Carrot with chive

Mix 3.5oz (100g) of grated carrots with 1.1oz (30g) of finely chopped chive; add 1 tablespoon of vegetable oil and put some finely chopped cucumber on top.

Blood-cleansing salad

Grate 1.8oz (50g) of beets and 1.8oz (50g) g of carrots; add 1.8oz (50g) of chopped cabbage, 1.5 tablespoon of olive oil, and 1.5 tablespoons of honey. Mix everything well and put a cupful of berries or red currant on top.

Cabbage with cumin

Chop up finely 3.5oz (100g) of cabbage; add 1 tablespoon of honey and 1 teaspoon of ground cumin

Tomatoes with carrot and nuts or biscuits

Crush 3.5oz (100g) of tomatoes and mix with 3.5oz (100g) of grated carrots, 1.1oz (30g) of chopped parsley, and 1.8oz (50g) of ground nuts or biscuits. Add 1.5 tablespoon of olive oil and mix again.

Tomatoes stuffed with sauerkraut

Cut off the top of a tomato (3-4mm) and carve out its inside, leaving only the wall 3-4mm thick. Mix the inside with finely chopped red sauerkraut and 1 teaspoon of plant oil, and stuff the tomato with this mixture. Put 1 teaspoon of mayonnaise or whipped cream on top, together with some chopped parsley or green onions.

Salad from green beans

Remove the fibers from 2.1oz (60g) of young and tender bean pods and chop the pods finely. Add 1.8oz (50g) of lettuce chopped into larger pieces and 2 tablespoons of sunflower oil (you can also add 1 teaspoon of honey for better taste).

Carrot and celery

Mix 1.8oz (50g) of grated carrot with 1.8oz (50g) of chopped celery, grated 1 of a cucumber, 1.8oz (50g) of ground nuts, and 1 tablespoon of honey. (You can use 2 tablespoons of sunflower oil instead of nuts.)

Leek salad

Chop finely 2oz (60g) of leek, add 3 tablespoons of mayonnaise, let it stand for 1 hour, and then add 1 tablespoon of chopped celery, 1 pinch of cumin, and 1 teaspoon of honey dissolved in 2 teaspoons of water.

Pumpkin salad

Grate a carrot, 1.8oz (50g) of pumpkin, and 0.9oz (25g) of celery. Add 0.9oz (25g) of chopped chive or red onion and 1 ground nut.

Winter salads

Beets and nuts

Grate a cooked large beet and 0.5 of a raw small beet. Add 1 crushed garlic clove and 1 tablespoons of vegetable oil. Mix everything well and put some ground nuts and a pinch of chopped chive on top.

Potato salad

Mix 2.6oz (75g) of finely chopped potato with 1.8oz (50g) of ground nuts, 1 tablespoon of honey, and 1 teaspoon of grated horseradish.

Vitamin-rich salad

Grate 1.8oz (50g) of carrots, 2.6oz (75g) of cabbage, and 1.8oz (50g) of potatoes. Add 0.9oz (25g) of chopped parsley, 0.9oz (25g) of leek, 2 tablespoons of vegetable oil, 1 tablespoon of honey, and 1.8oz (50g) of ground nuts. Mix everything well.

Carrot and horseradish salad

Grate a large carrot and 1.8oz (50g) of celery roots. Add 1 tablespoon of grated horseradish, 0.35oz (10g) of ground nuts, and 1 tablespoon of vegetable oil. Mix everything well.

Holiday salad

Take a small red or white cabbage 2.6oz (75g) and chop it finely. Add 0.5 of a grated average-sized carrot, 0.5 of a pickled cucumber, a 4-inch/10cm long finely chopped leek stem, 5 ground walnuts, 1 tablespoon of vegetable oil, and 3 tablespoons of oat cereal. Mix everything well.

Sauces and mayonnaises

Store-bought sauces and mayonnaises usually contain preservatives, coloring agents, and other substances foreign for our body and polluting our blood. This is why it is a good idea to prepare them on our own.

Lemon oil

Gradually add juice from 1 or 2 lemons as you stir 0.9oz (25g) of vegetable oil.

Nut mayonnaise (best prepared directly before the meal)

Mix 2 tablespoons of ground nuts with 1 teaspoon of vegetable oil to make a thick pulp. Then add 3-4 tablespoons of vegetable oil and whip it while gradually adding juice squeezed from 1 lemon.

Cream sauce

Mix juice from 0.5 lemon with 3 tablespoons of cream. Add a crushed garlic clove, 0.5 teaspoon of finely chopped chive or grated onion, and 1 tablespoon of vegetable oil. Mix everything well.

Tomato sauce

Mix 6 parts of vegetable oil with 1 part of lemon juice. Blend it with tomato juice and add some grated celery for better taste.

"Rainbow" - a vitamin-rich mayonnaise

Whip 2 egg yolks while slowly adding 3 tablespoons of vegetable oil. Mix it with 1 tablespoon of grated celery or 1 teaspoon of grated onion and add some lemon juice. Whip well until it reaches normal mayonnaise thickness. You can color it green (with spinach juice), orange (with carrot juice), or pink (with red currant juice).

Cold soups

Cold soups are the most suitable on hot days of summer and fall. People who have trouble with regular bowel movement are recommended to eat them all year long. They are very beneficial for our health because, unlike hot soups, they preserve all vitamins, minerals, structured water, and oxygen contained in their ingredients.

Tomato and cucumber soup

Pour 10 tablespoons of sour milk on 3 tablespoons of oat cereal and let it stand for 2-3 hours. Add some grated cucumbers, chopped tomatoes, and 1 crushed garlic clove, then mix everything well and put some chopped parsley on top.

Tomato soup with cream

Mix 2 grated tomatoes with 1 tablespoon of cream, pour the mixture on 3 tablespoons of oat cereal, let it stand for 1 hour, and add some chopped parsley.

Raspberry (or wild strawberry) soup

To 1 cup of sour milk add 3 tablespoons of mineral water and 3 tablespoons of crushed raspberries (or wild strawberries). You can also add 1 tablespoon of honey.

Soup from dried fruits

Soak overnight (8-10 hours) a handful of dried fruits (plums, raisins, apples, or pears), strain, add 2 tablespoons of oat cereal and 1 tablespoon of honey, let it stand for another 3-5 hours, and eat for breakfast or dinner.

Desserts

Apple snow

Grate 2 or 3 apples and add 1 tablespoon of honey dissolved in 1 tablespoon of water. Mix it well. Separately, whip 2 egg whites while slowly adding some lemon juice. Mix everything together and whip again. Finally, you can decorate it with canned peaches, pears, frozen strawberries, fresh raspberries, or currants (use your imagination).

Apple web

Whip 2 egg yolks and 2 egg whites separately. Mix them and whip again. Dissolve 1 tablespoon of honey in 1 tablespoons of warm water. Grate 3 sweet apples and add 2 teaspoons of lemon juice to them. Mix everything together and whip again. Decorate with fresh fruits - berries, chunks of orange or grapefruit.

Honey cake

Mix 1.05oz (30 g) of lemon juice with 2.1oz (60g) of ground walnuts or peanuts. Let it stand for half an hour, and then add 2 tablespoons of honey and 2.1oz (60g) of ground rice. Mix everything and form into cakes. Put some ground roasted sunflower seeds on top.

INDEX

A

Abdomen, 109, 194, 210
Acetic acid, 150
Aging, 24, 35, 74, 125, 171
AIDS, 123
Alcoholism, treating 173-179
Anemia, 37, 39, 87, 150, 176
  remedies against, 179-180
Antibiotics, 47, 116, 140, 155
  natural, 120, 191
Anxiety, 73, 77, 196
Apple juice, 96
  liver cleanse with, 149-150
Apple cider vinegar, 111, 155,
  215
  making of, 153
  therapies, 150-152, 190,
  191, 211
Arrhythmia, remedy against,
  180
Arteriosclerosis, 85, 89, 147
  treating, 180-181
Arthritis, 36, 45, 94
  remedies against, 69, 70,
  182
Ascaris (intestinal parasites),
  remedies against, 182, 183
Ascorbic acids, 40
Aspirin, 47, 156, 185
Asthma, 10, 31, 104, 105
  remedies against, 185
Autotoxication, 103, 105

B

Back pain, 36, 45-71, 87, 104,
133
Baldness, 163-169
Baths, 32, 33, 48, 59, 61, 100
Beet juice, 95, 96, 97, 111,
  179, 181, 192, 198, 208,
  211
Black radish remedies, 31, 32,
68, 180, 185, 202, 204, 206
Bladder, 27
  treating bladder stones, 202
Bloating, 150, 183-184
Blood pressure, 39, 80, 96
  high, 39, 147, 152, 198
  low, 77, 96, 207, 208
  normalize, 142, 208
  reduce, 78, 126, 198
Boils, (furuncles), 193